AEROBIC FITNESS

JOHN MASON

Kangaroo Press

AEROBIC FITNESS

First published in Australia in 1999 by Kangaroo Press
An imprint of Simon & Schuster (Australia) Pty Limited
20 Barcoo Street, East Roseville NSW 2069

A Viacom Company
Sydney New York London Toronto Tokyo Singapore

National Library of Australia
Cataloguing-in-Publication data

Mason, John. 1951– .
   Aerobic fitness.

   Bibliography.
   Includes index.
   ISBN 0 86417 960 X.

   1. Aerobic exercises. 2. Exercise. 3. Physical fitness.
   I. Title.

613.71

Cover design:	Anna Soo Design
Cover photograph:	Running Bear Australia Pty Ltd
Text and photographs:	John Mason
Illustrations:	Lorenzo Lucia (based on sketches by Stephen Mason and Amanda Moss)
Additional photographs:	No Fear, Only Fitness (Australia) Pty Ltd, Running Bare Australia Pty Ltd, Workout Workshop Gymnasium Equipment
Editorial assistants:	Lyn Quirk, Reg. Fitness Leader, M.Ed, Dip.Nutrition, Dip.Nat.Therapies Kerryn Cormick, B.App.Sci.–Phys.Ed., Grad.Dip. Sport Mgt., Reg. Fitness Leader Iain Harrison, Dip.Hort.Sc. Paul Plant, B.App.Sci., Cert. Massage
Design and typesetting:	Midland Typesetters, Maryborough

Set in 9/12 Palatino.
Printed in Hong Kong by Colourcraft

10 9 8 7 6 5 4 3 2 1

CONTENTS

PREFACE

Aerobic fitness contributes more to your quality of life than perhaps any other aspect of fitness. A person with reasonable aerobic fitness usually has a healthy heart, lungs and circulatory system. This means that they are able to breathe well, absorb plenty of oxygen into the blood, and efficiently transfer that oxygen throughout the body. It also means that waste products can be easily removed from the body by being absorbed into the blood and carried effectively to where they can be eliminated.

A key ingredient for ensuring a long life is maintaining a healthy body and mind. By maintaining good aerobic fitness you will generally perform better in intellectual as well as physical pursuits; you will tend to resist illness better, live longer and find it easier to maintain a healthy mental state.

This book will assist the reader to generally improve their aerobic fitness levels and overall health. It looks at equipment, facilities and current trends within the fitness industry, including fitness testing, exercises, programming and safety. One chapter discusses the special exercise requirements of pregnant women, older adults, children, overweight individuals and people with disabilities and/or health problems. The reader will learn about the body and its functions, enabling them to educate others to reach their aerobic potential.

INTRODUCTION

Staying aerobically fit

To remain aerobically fit you need to regularly participate in activities which increase your heart-rate above its normal level. This could be exercise but it could also be work; in fact it can be any physical activity that causes the heart to beat faster than normal. For this activity to be effective, the heart-rate must be sustained at a raised level for at least 20 minutes in each session, and there must be at least three such sessions each week. If the raised heart-rate is to be sustained for 20 minutes, the session probably needs to go for at least 30 minutes, allowing time for the heart-rate to gradually increase at the beginning of the session, and to gradually decrease at the end.

A modern epidemic

The lack of aerobic fitness is in many ways a problem fostered by modern living.

If you are not physically active at work or in your leisure, this may result in problems with aerobic fitness. If you find physical activity such as climbing stairs or going for long walks difficult, and if you are also overweight or frequently stressed, then you need to consider paying more attention to your aerobic fitness, perhaps as a matter of urgency. It is recommended that a medical clearance be obtained before beginning any exercise routine.

What can you do?

Regular exercise will improve aerobic fitness. Perhaps attending classes at the gym, jogging or walking regularly. Playing sport is another option, but remember, you need three sessions a week—so playing sport once a week is not sufficient, even if it is for a couple of hours. Many people find organised, regular exercise options very difficult to commit to. If that is the

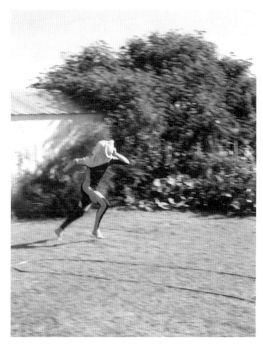

A quick, energetic sprint is mainly an anaerobic exercise.

case for you, there are lots of other options which can be equally beneficial—remember, anything that raises the heart-rate continuously can be effective. Consider working in the garden, taking up a part-time job that involves physical activity, playing with your children more often; if you don't have children of your own, consider becoming a scout or guide leader and getting active with a group of teenagers.

The difference between aerobic and anaerobic exercise

Anaerobic exercises concentrate on movements that require no, or minimal, oxygen. They are quick, explosive actions that often last no more

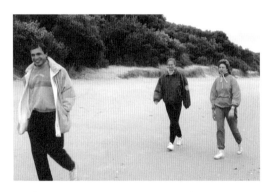

Walking on the beach can be an excellent aerobic activity for any age. It is less energetic than a quick sprint, but will raise and sustain the heart-rate above its normal resting level.

than one and a half to two minutes. Anaerobic exercises concentrate on improving the strength, speed and power of muscular movements.

During the first two minutes of exercise, the body cannot get enough oxygen to supply the heart and muscles (which need to work faster than normal). This is referred to as 'oxygen debt'. Once the heart and lungs increase their activity, however, they are providing oxygen faster than normal to the body, allowing aerobic activity to supply sufficient energy for movement.

Anaerobic exercise utilises an energy-rich molecule, adenosine triphosphate (ATP), and creatine phosphate (CP) already stored in the muscles to meet initial energy requirements. Energy demand then switches to the aerobic system, where the body can use and deliver oxygen to the muscles. The body therefore cannot work in a fast or powerful manner for longer than two minutes because of its need for oxygen. This first phase of exercise gives a quick rise in heart-rate.

Aerobic exercises focus on making heart and respiration rates work more efficiently; in so doing they improve cardiorespiratory fitness.

If the heart-rate increases to a certain level and remains there, the aerobic energy system is predominant. Muscles are generally moved repeatedly and for a longer period of time during aerobic exercise, when the body requires more oxygen which must be breathed in to allow it to travel to the muscles through the blood. Aerobic exercise normally burns the carbohydrates already stored in the blood as glucose, and in the muscles and liver as glycogen, to meet energy needs, and then resorts to burning fat to supply energy. The aerobic system usually commences after approximately one minute and can continue for up to an hour or longer.

Examples of aerobic and anaerobic exercises

Anaerobic exercises are high energy, short in duration, usually flat-out, and rely on stored fuel. The 100-metre sprint, shot put and high jump are all good examples. Aerobic exercise is continuous, like cycling, swimming and walking. (Even sitting and reading a book is aerobic, because the body is breathing at a constant rate which can be maintained.) The more intense an aerobic activity the greater the level of fitness that can be achieved.

It can be said that aerobic classes such as those commonly run at a gymnasium are not just aerobic, because of the varied intensity of the different exercises. Participants may well find themselves doing anaerobic-type exercises at some stages during the class. This provides variety and enables other aspects of fitness to be improved as well, including muscular strength and endurance.

Chapter 1 explains the biology of aerobic fitness, allowing the reader to understand the process of making and utilising energy. This physiology will define and relate concepts, enabling the reader to better increase their aerobic fitness.

CHAPTER 1

THE BIOLOGY OF AEROBIC FITNESS

Aerobic fitness can be calculated at any time during a person's life. It is assumed that a younger person will have better aerobic fitness than an older person—this is not always true, however. Additionally, it is possible to improve aerobic fitness over time.

To achieve optimum aerobic development it helps to understand some of the principles that govern aerobic fitness and aerobic capacity.

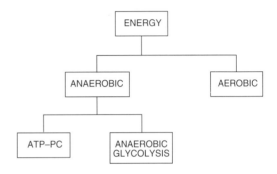

Aerobic capacity
Aerobic capacity is determined by an individual's ability to extract and utilise oxygen. This measurement is termed VO_2max; at rest the body utilises 3.5 millilitres of oxygen per kilogram of body weight per minute to sustain life.

Athletes have recorded VO_2max scores in the vicinity of 90 ml/kg/min. An average middle-aged male with poor fitness may score about 26 ml/kg/min. When physical fitness and the capacity of the heart improves, VO_2max will increase.

Fatigue occurs when the body cannot perform to its optimal capacity, either physically or mentally.

The human body requires energy to perform physical functions. This energy is derived from food sources—carbohydrates, fats and proteins. Energy-releasing reactions break down food for the production of energy.

An ATP (adenosine triphosphate) molecule is an energy-rich molecule made up of adenosine and three phosphate groups. When ATP is broken down to adenosine diphosphate or ADP (two phosphates) and a free phosphate molecule, energy is released. ATP provides energy for muscles to contract maximally for about 15 seconds. This energy system is used for short bursts of intense energy.

SOURCES OF ATP

ATP can be supplied to the body in three ways:

- Anaerobically through the ATP–PC system
- Anaerobically through anaerobic glycolysis
- Through the aerobic system.

ATP–PC SYSTEM

This system supplies instant energy. Only about 85 grams of ATP is stored in the muscle at any one time, enough to allow between one and 10 seconds of explosive activity to occur. As rapidly as these energy supplies are broken down, they are restored, to the extent of 50 per cent within 30 seconds and 100 per cent in two or three minutes.

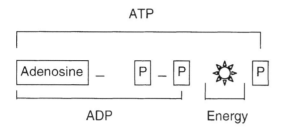

This can continue, allowing the body to repeat short bursts of activity; however, if an activity requires repeated muscular contractions for longer than 10 seconds, the energy must be sourced from other stores.

ANAEROBIC GLYCOLYSIS

This energy comes from the breakdown of stored glycogen in the muscles where pyruvic acid is formed, then ATP. This process occurs with events lasting between 10 and 90 seconds. Anaerobic glycolysis, working in the absence of oxygen, produces a by-product called lactic acid. This lactic acid builds up in the muscles and blood and causes fatigue.

Once this lactic acid is produced (after approximately 55 seconds of flat-out exercise) it takes about 45–60 minutes for it to be removed and for the athlete to be completely recovered. Removal of lactic acid occurs in the presence of oxygen via the bloodstream. Light walking or jogging will assist in this removal.

The extra oxygen available is called 'oxygen debt', which simply refers to having more oxygen than required, and acts as a reserve for a runner or football player to use in the last-second sprint for the finish line or the ball.

After completion of exercise, there may be a lactic acid build-up in the muscles, which needs to be removed to help reduce soreness.

LACTIC ACID SYSTEM

When a maximal effort is continued beyond the extent of the phosphate energy system, energy is provided from glycogen stored in the muscles. In this system glucose (or glycogen) goes through various chemical processes to produce ATP plus lactic acid. One glucose molecule is broken down into carbon dioxide and water, and in turn produces two ATP molecules. The amount of ATP produced this way is small. This is a more complex procedure using only carbohydrates as fuel, and not requiring oxygen for the process.

The energy produced by the lactic acid system is used, for example, in 400-metre track races and 100-metre swimming events. Continuous activities which lead to exhaustion in 45–50 seconds result in maximal values for lactic acid accumulation, which can affect blood pH. Blood pH should be around 7.3, and never drop below 6.8. Normally, however, the lactic acid system is self-limiting, and should not develop such problems. Generally the result will be a feeling of fatigue which will cause an athlete (or someone doing heavy bursts of work) to slow down. Once lactic acid is produced, it requires 45 to 60 minutes to be removed from the body, and for the athlete to recover.

AEROBIC SYSTEM

This system, which we use every day for living, is very important. It is also the predominant system for marathon runners and long–distance events. Any activity lasting longer than two minutes will utilise the aerobic system.

Glycogen becomes the preferred source of fuel because more energy is derived from the breakdown of glucose per litre of oxygen. One molecule of sugar can produce 36 ATP. The by-products of this system are carbon dioxide and water.

The equation summarising the aerobic energy system is:

$$C_6H_{12}O_6 + 6O_2 \longrightarrow 6CO_2 + 6H_2O + energy$$

This formula is a simple glucose molecule ($C_6H_{12}O_6$) oxidised to produce carbon dioxide (CO_2) which is respired out of the body, water (H_2O) and energy. The energy is used to convert ADP to ATP.

The aerobic system involves the formation of carbon dioxide plus water plus ATP, from fats, proteins and/or carbohydrates, in the presence of oxygen, to produce large amounts of ATP.

This system is more complex than the ATP–PC system, but the only limiting factor is usually the supply of oxygen.

The body will normally try to use this system, and only use other systems to produce ATP if oxygen is in short supply. A shortage of oxygen can occur when activity first starts, or when activity is placing higher demands for oxygen than can be supplied by breathing.

> The oxygen system is an **aerobic system**.
>
> The ATP–PC (phosphate) and lactic acid systems are **anaerobic systems**.
>
> The body uses anaerobic systems for energy supply *only* when the aerobic system cannot meet the demand.
>
> *Example*
> In a person running a marathon, where breathing is not supplying sufficient oxygen to produce ATP through the aerobic system, the lactic acid system may start to be used, resulting in a build-up of lactic acid; *or* the ATP–PC (phosphate) system may be used, resulting in a depletion of phosphocreatine in the muscles.

At the completion of exercise, there may be a lactic acid build up in the body which must be removed. Lactic acid removal requires the expenditure of further energy which must be supplied aerobically; thus extra oxygen may be required. This extra oxygen requirement after exercise is called the 'oxygen debt'.

Excessive exercising may result in a participant reaching the point called 'hitting the wall'. This occurs when a skeletal muscle or group of muscles loses strength or gets progressively weaker due to insufficient oxygen, deletion of glycogen, or a build-up of lactic acid.

ENERGY AND CALORIES

Energy is usually expressed as calories, which is the term most people associate with weight loss and exercise.

The table on page 4 illustrates different activities and its calorie expenditure.

Further details on energy and its measurements can be found in Appendix I.

WHAT HAPPENS DURING EXERCISE

As exercise starts:

- Heart rate and respiration rate increase
- VO$_2$max increases
- Lactate initially increases
- RQ drops at first, then increases.

As intensity of exercise increases, the use of fat decreases; at 50 per cent VO$_2$max, fat use can reach zero.

BREATHING

During aerobic exercise the oxygen supply to the body must be optimised. For this to happen, two things are important:

- The way you breathe
- The quality of the air you breathe in.

By optimising the oxygen supply:

- Lung elasticity increases
- Blood volume increases
- Heart performance improves
- Circulation of blood becomes better
- Cell metabolism improves, hence muscle performance is better and waste products are removed more efficiently from the cells
- The likelihood of hyperventilation during exercise is lower.

The way you breathe

Consider how you breathe and its impact on your health.

Type of activity	Description	Kilocalories per hour
Sedentary	listening to music Stationary–little or no movement, e.g. sitting, watching TV,	80–100
Light	Slow walking, light housework, cooking	110–160
Moderate	Medium walking, mopping, sweeping, light gardening	170–240
Vigorous	Heavy housework, fast walking, general gardening, golfing	250–350
Strenuous	Running, tennis, football, cycling, dancing	350 or more

Modified from Robinson et al. (1986) *Normal and Therapeutic Nutrition*, Macmillan, New York

- *Deep or shallow?* Deep breathing is considered better for overall health.
- *Slow or fast?* Slow breathing is important when the body is relaxed.
- *Through the nose or mouth?* Breathing through the nose utilises the natural filtration system of the nasal passages.

The quality of the air you breathe

Consider the quality of the air you breathe and how this may affect health.

- *Air conditioning?* Air-conditioning units can spread air borne sicknesses.
- *Pollen, dust, allergens?* Allergies to these and other items impede breathing in many people.
- *Vegetation?* Oxygen levels are higher around vegetation. Fresh air is important to all, especially in those activities where oxygen is crucial. It is important to consider allergies and asthma.
- *High altitude?* High altitude pre-season training allows athletes to increase the oxygen in their blood. However, oxygen levels become lower as altitude increases.

Oxygen

There is some evidence to indicate that holding the breath just prior to an exercise (e.g. taking a deep breath before swimming the first few strokes) may actually increase performance. However, it can be dangerous in some cases, like swimming, where 'shallow water blackout' may occur (a type of fainting under water), possibly resulting in drowning.

Breathing oxygen-enriched air during exercise can be beneficial through:

- Increased endurance capacity
- Lower heart-rate (during sub-optimum work)
- Lower accumulation of lactic acid
- Lower breathing rate.

Oxygen availability decreases with altitude, hence the likelihood of peak performance decreases at higher altitudes. Although oxygen is sometimes administered to athletes during recovery, research does not tend to support this having any significant benefit under normal conditions.

TRAINING RESPONSE

Different people will respond in different ways to the same training stimulus. The *form* of the response to training does, however, remain the same for everyone. There are several stages in the response, and each stage is modified by several different factors. When you understand the form of a training response, and the modifiers, you can then devise training programs which give results as close as possible to the desired effect.

The stages in the training response are:

1. Tolerance capacity
2. Fatigue
3. Recovery
4. Training effect (or over-compensation)
5. Deterioration.

Tolerance capacity In the first part of training, performance is generally adequate or perhaps better than adequate. In this phase, the person can tolerate the demands of training without excessive stress. Modifiers which affect the duration of this stage include the level of exertion and the mental and physical condition of the person exercising.

Fatigue When a person begins to exercise beyond their capacity, their level of performance (perhaps measured by the quantity of energy being burnt) will start to deteriorate. The fatigue phase begins when this deterioration starts to occur. A person is in the fatigue phase when unable to produce an adequate response (i.e. perform a task to an expected optimum level). The severity of training is a significant modifier affecting the duration of this stage.

Recovery This phase commences once exercise stops, or is reduced to a very low level, allowing energy reserves to again build, and performance potential to start increasing.

Training effect Once energy reserves have returned to 'normal' they tend to continue building for a short time (over-compensation). The net result is a slight increase on the energy reserves available prior to exercise. Properly designed training provides time for recovery and over-compensation to occur.

Deterioration The training effect is in the main a temporary effect; without repeated exercise (and repeated training effects) there will be a 'decay' over time.

With regular exercise, training effects can accumulate and performance potential can be increased—this is the basis for exercise programming.

FATIGUE WHILE EXERCISING

Fatigue during exercise tends to occur in three stages, generally in the same sequence.

1. *Depletion of performance in the central nervous system*—this can affect behaviour, performance quality, and efficiency of movement. This is seen in the person's attitude or mood, as well as in their actions. They may still be able to perform, but their mood may change from happy to a more serious or even negative mood. They may acknowledge difficulty as the first threshold is approached.

2. *Depletion of energy reserves*—this reduces the capacity to perform. This is indicated by a deterioration in performance (e.g. distance being run, amount of weight being lifted, times being clocked/rate of activity). A higher level of activity may be sustained by using extra muscles, or an extra psychological effort, but performance efficiency will decrease (that is, more energy will be used to perform the same tasks if they are being carried out by 'alternative' muscles).

3. *Morphological changes*—this can change the state of the blood and cause tissue damage. The fact that this stage has been reached may be indicated by incomplete recovery between repetitions (e.g. in lifting weights); progressive deterioration in performance despite deeper (heavier) breathing (this can indicate lactic acid build up); distressed behaviour.

   Note: The nervous system will normally deteriorate well before any morphological deterioration; thus the condition of the nervous system should be the main factor in determining training loads.

   On any indication of this third stage being reached, all activity should immediately cease.

FATIGUE BETWEEN TRAINING SESSIONS

If there is inadequate rest between training sessions, there will be inadequate recovery. This must be avoided. Such a state may be indicated by:

- Negative attitude or mood
- Any abnormal psychological behaviour

- Withdrawal
- Reluctance to commence another exercise session
- Warm-up activity poorer than normal
- Muscle fatigue or soreness
- Higher than normal pulse rate during rest period
- Sore throat or flu symptoms
- Feelings of discomfort
- Feeling sick or nauseous
- Dizziness.

RECOVERY FROM EXERCISE

Metabolic pathways involved in the transition from exercise to rest are different to those involved from rest to exercise. The purpose of the recovery phase is to return the body to its pre-exercise condition. To do this the body must:

- Replenish energy stores depleted by exercise
- Remove any build-up of lactic acid (lactates).

As exercise slows:

- Energy demand decreases
- Oxygen consumption continues at a higher than normal level for the first two or three minutes following exercise. After this oxygen consumption declines slowly to near pre-exercise levels. Here the term 'oxygen debt' describes any excess of oxygen consumed during recovery over that normally consumed at rest. Oxygen debt is *not* simply the oxygen required to replace oxygen stores which were used during exercise. In fact very little oxygen from the muscles needs replacing. It is the sources of energy (ATP, PC and glycogen) which need to be replenished, and oxygen is needed to fuel this replenishment.

Alactacid oxygen debt component

This refers to the rapid breathing phase in perhaps the first two or three minutes following exercise. During this period the oxygen debt is used to replenish muscular stores of ATP and PC. The alactacid debt may range from 2 to 2.5

litres over that timeframe, which can vary according to the exercises and activities undertaken.

Lactacid oxygen debt component

This is the slower phase of recovery where oxygen consumption gradually decreases. Lactic acid is removed in this phase. This phase is about 30 times slower than the alactacid phase, because it takes longer to metabolise lactic acid and restore phosphagens. Light exercise will, however, speed up this phase.

Consuming high carbohydrate foods within 30 minutes of exercise is said to be one of the best ways to restore or top up glycogen levels. Muscle glycogen stores take up to 72 hours to completely restore after aerobic exercise and are affected largely by diet. Eating a banana or a similar high carbohydrate food straight after exercising will assist with the next endurance session undertaken.

It has been common in the past for endurance athletes to carbohydrate-load prior to a major event. This involves depleting muscle glycogen stores a week before the race by exercising hard and eating a low carbohydrate diet. After several days of this the body is rested and loaded up on a high carbohydrate/low fat diet. For the event glycogen stores are topped up completely by providing the body with quantities of high carbohydrate fuels. This method, however, has caused much concern in medical circles due to the dizzy spells, headaches, nausea, and in some athletes a disturbance in heart rhythm, occurring in the initial stages. So even though carbohydrate loading looks like a good way of ensuring high carbohydrate levels for an event, it is now suggested by some authorities that the same result can be achieved by eating a low fat/high carbohydrate diet all the time. Practising carbohydrate loading is potentially dangerous; if athletes insist on doing it they must have some carbohydrates in their diet when initially depleting to prevent the side effects mentioned.

Lactic acid

About 10 per cent of the lactic acid removed from the muscles during recovery is converted to glucose; 75 per cent is oxidised in the presence of oxygen to produce CO_2 and O_2, while the remainder is unaccounted for. A gradual cooling down following exercise (rather than an abrupt stop) will eliminate lactic acid retention. Excessive lactic acid remaining in the muscles can cause pain.

TIME OF DAY TO EXERCISE

A number of studies* have indicated that the aerobic system works better in the afternoon than in the morning, therefore optimum performance is more likely in the afternoon. The reasons for this optimum performance are numerous—for example, the activity of metabolism, warmth and stretching of muscles, mentally alertness to physical exercise. Thus exercise classes and competitive events are best scheduled after midday.

To gain optimum peak physical performance it is best to train at a time comparable to the time at which a professional athlete would be performing, e.g. train for a marathon at the same time of day as the actual marathon will occur.

HUMAN ANATOMY

An understanding of basic human anatomy is an important part of understanding how the body moves during activity, which exercises are best for exercising different parts of the body, and which exercises are potentially dangerous. Readers are referred to Appendix II on page 114, for a detailed discussion of the skeletal system.

MUSCULAR SYSTEM

Parts of a muscle

Tendons A band of connective tissue attaching bone to muscle.

* *Journal of Sports Medicine*, Vol. 36, No. 3, 1996

Deep fascia A layer of connective tissue surrounding a muscle and holding it in position. It is dense tissue and lines the body wall.
Epimysium The layer of tissue enclosing or covering a bundle of muscle tissue, i.e. covering a whole muscle.
Perimysium Connective tissue covering bundles of 10 to 100 muscle fibres.
Muscle fibre A collection of muscle cells which responds by movement when stimulated.
Sarcolemma The cell membrane of muscle fibre (particularly relevant in skeletal muscle).
Endomysium Tissue inside a fascicle between the individual muscle fibre inside the perimysium.
Fascicle A bundle of muscle fibres including the perimysium and all enclosed by it.
Motor neuron A neuron that transmits nerve impulses from the brain or central nervous system to the glands or muscles that respond to the impulse.
Blood vessel Carries blood to and from the muscle tissue.

How muscles move (the simple version)

Muscles move both by contraction, where they shorten in length, and by relaxation, where they increase in length. During contraction, thick and thin muscle filaments slide past each other inwards towards the centre of the muscle.

Muscle fibre (filament) types

There are three types of muscle filament.

Thick filaments These are around 16 nm (nanometres) in diameter, and are made up 44 per cent of the protein myosin. They form cross-bridges between thin filaments. When contraction occurs, the cross-bridges move the thin filaments together.

Elastic filaments These are less than 1 nm in diameter and 9 per cent made up of the protein titin. They anchor the thick filaments and help stabilise them during contraction.

Thin filaments These are around 8 nm in diameter and contain three different proteins (22 per cent actin, 5 per cent tropomyosin, 5 per cent troponin). They slide along the thick filaments during contraction.

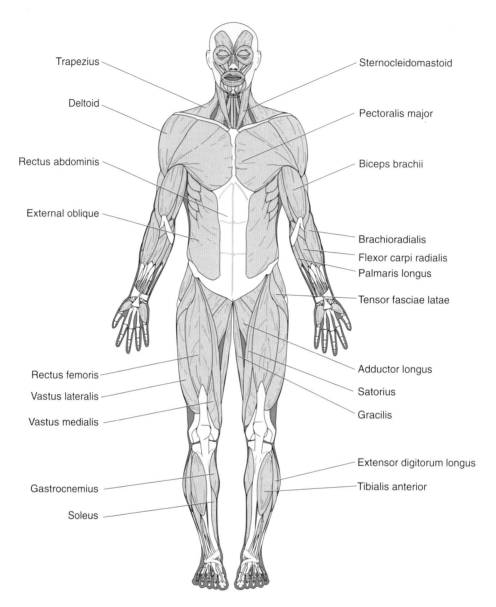

Trapezius — Sternocleidomastoid

Deltoid — Pectoralis major

Rectus abdominis — Biceps brachii

External oblique — Brachioradialis
— Flexor carpi radialis
— Palmaris longus

— Tensor fasciae latae

Rectus femoris — Adductor longus

Vastus lateralis — Satorius

Vastus medialis — Gracilis

Gastrocnemius — Extensor digitorum longus
— Tibialis anterior

Soleus

Muscle types

Three kinds of muscle are found in the body: smooth (or involuntary) muscle; striated (skeletal or voluntary) muscle; and cardiac muscle.

Smooth muscle

Found in the walls of the intestines, in the urogenital system and in the blood vessels. It is called 'involuntary' because it works automatically, without any conscious effort being required. It cannot be stopped or started at will.

A good example of this kind of movement is peristalsis, the muscular contractions and relaxations which move food down the oesophagus and through the small and large intestines. Smooth muscle is made up of elongated, spindle-shaped cells with the nucleus placed in the middle of the cell.

Striated muscle

Skeletal, striated or voluntary muscle is the type of muscle found in the arms and legs which can

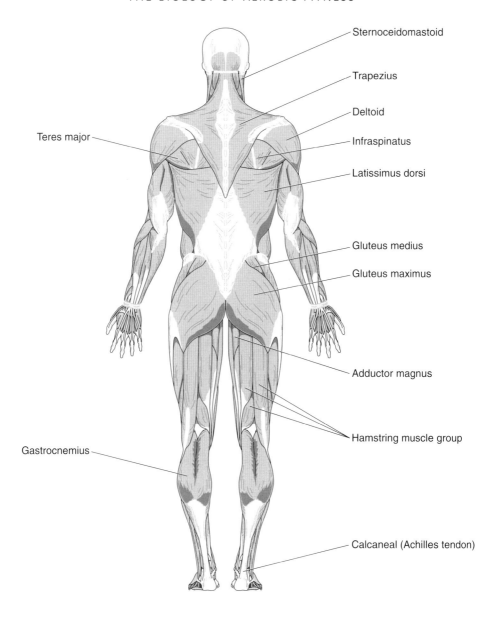

Sternoceidomastoid

Trapezius

Deltoid

Infraspinatus

Latissimus dorsi

Teres major

Gluteus medius

Gluteus maximus

Adductor magnus

Hamstring muscle group

Gastrocnemius

Calcaneal (Achilles tendon)

be rested at will. Skeletal muscle is made up of striated muscle fibres (of three different types) supported by connective tissues attached to bone by tendons or an aponeurosis (a broad flat extension layer of tendon), and stimulated by nerves. Each fibre is a muscle cell. Each fibre has many nuclei positioned near the surface of the cell.

Each individual muscle cell is made up of smaller fibres called myofibrils (*myo*- meaning 'muscle' in Greek). The sheath called the sarcolemma holds the myofibrils in a bundle, connects the muscle cell to tendons and gives elasticity. Each muscle fibre is controlled and activated by a branch from a motor neuron from the nervous system.

Under a powerful electron microscope, bands can be seen on each myofibril. This consists of very fine filaments of two proteins, actin and myosin. It is believed that the actin filaments slide together during the contraction of the muscle, so that neither the actin nor the myosin filaments actually change their lengths.

The contraction of muscles is a positive action requiring the use of energy. When you pick up a brick, for example, the muscles of the arm and fingers contract as you grip the brick and the arm muscles contract as you lift the brick upwards. You can drop the brick by relaxing the arm and finger muscles. Throwing the brick requires more contraction of the muscles and a greater supply of energy. This energy is supplied as a result of a number of chemical reactions which take place inside the muscles.

One such reaction is the breakdown of adenosine triphosphatase (ATP) as discussed on page 1. The protein filaments of myosin act as an enzyme to break down ATP to ADP (adenosine diphosphatase) and phosphoric acid. This reaction releases a great deal of energy which is used by the muscle fibres to cause contraction. As long as ATP is being broken down the muscle remains active, but when this reaction stops, the muscle becomes relaxed. Another reaction is the breakdown of glycogen into lactic acid with the production of energy.

Cardiac muscle

This type of muscle is both striated and involuntary in nature. It differs from striated voluntary muscle in the following ways:

- The nuclei are placed in the centre of the cells
- The fibres branch out to form networks
- Between the cells are found membranes called intercalated discs
- Most importantly of all, cardiac muscle is not subject to fatigue in the way that striated voluntary muscle becomes tired and less effective.

Types of skeletal muscle fibre

There are three types of skeletal muscle fibres.

Slow oxidative type

Also called 'Type I', 'slow twitch' or 'fatigue resistant' fibres; characterised by:

- High numbers of blood capillaries (blood supply is good)
- A high capacity to generate ATP by aerobic system
- Splitting ATP at a slow rate, therefore they contract slowly
- High fatigue resistance.

Example: neck muscles.

Long distance runners tend to utilise slow twitch fibres which allow them to exercise for long periods before exhaustion.

Fast oxidative type

Also called 'Type IIA', 'fast twitch A' or 'fatiguable' fibres; characterised by:

- High numbers of blood capillaries (blood supply is good)
- High capacity to generate ATP by oxidative processes
- Splitting ATP at a very fast rate, hence muscles move fast
- Fatigue resistance, but not as resistant as slow oxidative fibres.

Example: leg muscles in sprinters.

Fast glycolytic type

Also called: 'Type IIB', 'fast twitch B' or 'fatiguable' fibres; characterised by:

- Fewer blood capillaries than the other types
- Contain a lot of glycogen
- Generation of ATP by glycolysis (an anaerobic process)
- Low fatigue resistance.

Example: arm muscles contain a lot of this type of fibre.

RESPIRATORY SYSTEM

The respiratory system consists of the trachea; two bronchi (singular = bronchus); two lungs; many alveolar sacs; many alveoli (singular = alveolus).

In the process of respiration oxygen in the air is taken into the body by way of the lungs and passed into the bloodstream; this is called inspiration. Carbon dioxide, one of the waste products from the production of energy, is carried by the bloodstream back to the lungs and expelled from the body; this is called expiration. The exchange of oxygen and carbon dioxide in the blood takes place in the tissues of the lungs.

The trachea is a tough tube of rings made of cartilage. The inside of the tube is lined with small, hair-like projections called cilia. Their function is to act as filters, screening the air drawn down into the lungs to remove particles of dust and foreign matter which are then swept up towards the mouth to be mixed with mucus. The cilia do this by continuously moving in wave-like, sweeping movements.

The trachea sits next to the oesophagus; because both food and air are drawn in at the mouth, the entrance to the trachea has to be closed when food is being swallowed to prevent food particles being carried into the lungs. The entrance is closed by the epiglottis, the small flap hanging down at the back of the throat. At its bottom end, the trachea divides into two smaller tubes called bronchi, which further subdivide into a structure known as the bronchial tree.

The bronchi, which are also made of tough, cartilage rings, lead one to each lung. Once inside the lungs, the bronchi divide into smaller and smaller branches called bronchioles, which in turn lead into small air sacs or alveolar sacs, consisting of many alveoli (*alveolus* means 'cavity' in Latin). The alveoli look very much like small balloons. Around each alveolus is a network of capillaries which connect the pulmonary artery blood vessels with those of the pulmonary vein.

The lungs are two cone-shaped, soft, spongy masses of tissue consisting of tubes and air sacs. Lungs are elastic and expand and contract as air is breathed in and out. The lungs are also well supplied with blood vessels which divide into many thread-like capillaries. The lungs lie within a special cavity in the body called the pleural cavity (*pleura* means 'rib' in Greek). Outside each lung is a slippery membrane called the pleural membrane which allows the lungs to slide more easily against the walls of the pleural cavity during breathing.

Physiology of respiration

The act of breathing is the result of the lungs expanding and contracting to draw air in and then push it out. The chest cavity, which contains the heart and lungs, is bounded on both sides by the ribs and at the bottom by the diaphragm, a

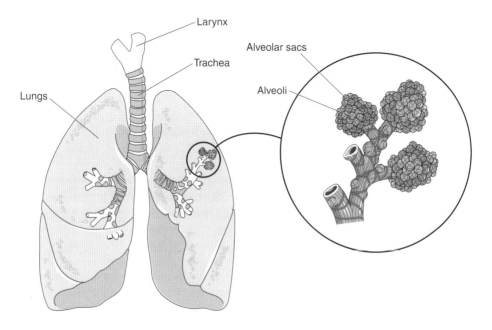

muscular plate which stretches from one side of the body to the other and divides the chest cavity from the abdominal cavity which contains the stomach and intestines.

Inside the chest cavity is a slight vacuum or negative pressure. By expanding the ribs outwards and pulling the diaphragm downwards, the size of the chest cavity is increased, the vacuum reduces, and the lungs can expand, pulling air in. This process is known as inspiration.

Try it for yourself. Take a deep breath and you will feel your ribs moving outwards. The whole movement, both of the ribs and the diaphragm, is muscular. When more air is needed, as in running, the muscles between the ribs work harder and expand the ribs further.

When both lungs have been filled with air, the diaphragm and ribs are relaxed and push inwards towards the lungs. This increases the vacuum inside the chest cavity by making it smaller. The lungs contract and push the air out in the process known as expiration.

Gaseous exchange

Blood which has been circulating through the body, which is now low in oxygen and high in carbon dioxide, is brought to the lungs by the pulmonary artery. This artery branches out and ends in capillaries surrounding the alveoli. The air in the alveoli, which has just been breathed in, is rich in oxygen.

A very rapid exchange now takes place. Oxygen passes through the thin walls of the alveoli into the capillaries while carbon dioxide passes in the opposite direction into the alveoli. The blood, now rich in oxygen, leaves the lungs through the pulmonary vein, which carries it to the heart from where it is pumped around the body and used up in the production of energy.

Rate and depth of breathing

Respiration is normally an involuntary movement which goes on without any conscious thought, although it can be voluntarily controlled for short periods, as when taking deep breaths, holding the breath and so on.

The rate and depth of breathing is controlled by the respiratory centre situated in the brain, which is stimulated by the levels of carbon dioxide in the blood. When the carbon dioxide level rises, the speed and depth of breathing is increased to expel it and increase the amount of oxygen available to replace it in the blood.

CIRCULATORY SYSTEM

The circulatory system consists of a network of vessels that circulate blood around the body. Included in the system is the heart, which acts as a pump. The vessels that carry blood away from the heart are called arteries and those that carry blood back to the heart are called veins. The blood carries oxygen and nutrients to the muscles and vital organs and carries carbon dioxide and waste products away. The circulatory system also includes the lymphatic system and the spleen. We will now look more closely at the importance of blood to the body.

Composition of blood

Blood is a fluid tissue consisting of red blood cells, platelets and white blood cells that move around the body in a fluid called plasma.

Plasma A straw-coloured fluid composed of 90 per cent water and 10 per cent solids. The solids are:

- Proteins: serum albumin, fibrinogen (concerned with blood clotting), globulin (deals with disease immunity)
- Hormones
- Lipids or fats
- Cholesterol
- Enzymes
- Inorganic chemicals (the ions of salts and acids, some of which are essential in cell metabolism and others which act as buffers, reducing strong acids and alkalis to weaker acids/alkalis and neutral salts)
- Nitrogenous compounds (amino acids, urea, uric acid and ammonium salts).

Red blood cells The red blood cells are called erythrocytes, and a single millilitre of blood contains 5 million of them. They are dish-shaped discs (concave on either side) which specialise in transporting oxygen. The oxygen is bound to a chemical called haemoglobin for transportation. The haemoglobin also gives blood its characteristic red colour.

Red blood cells, which are produced in the bone marrow, have a lifespan of three to four months. After that they disintegrate and the pigments produced by their destruction are excreted in bile.

Platelets Also called thrombocytes, these are small irregular-shaped fragments of protoplasm which are also formed in the bone marrow. They play an important role in the clotting of blood and the prevention of blood loss from wounds. They do this by sticking to each other and to the walls of blood vessels at the site of an injury. Platelets also release a substance called serotonin, which causes the blood vessels in the area of a wound to constrict in order to produce a drop in blood pressure.

White blood cells These are also called leucocytes; a single millilitre of blood contains between 4000 and 11 000. There are various types of leucocytes of different shapes and sizes. They play an extremely important part in the defence mechanism of the body. They can form barriers against disease and can also engulf harmful material such as bacteria. They play a role in the formation of antibodies and in the immune mechanism of the body. They are mostly formed in the bone marrow; some specialised types originate in the lymphatic tissues.

Functions of the blood

- To carry nutrients from the digestive tract to the body tissues and organs
- To carry oxygen from the lungs to the tissues and to carry carbon dioxide from the tissues back to the lungs
- To carry waste products from the tissues to the kidneys
- To carry hormones from the endocrine glands
- To regulate the body temperature by transporting heat from the deeper organs in the body up to the surface at the skin
- To maintain the water balance of the body
- To maintain the pH (acidity/alkalinity) balance of the tissues and organs
- To prevent too much blood loss by the ability of blood to clot
- To play an important part in the body's defence mechanism against disease.

Blood vessels

The blood travels through the body in an intricate network of tubes called blood vessels. The arrangement of the vessels allows blood to reach the furthermost corners of the body. Although the network is complicated, it is easy to understand if you remember that vessels carrying blood away from the heart are called arteries and vessels carrying blood towards the heart are called veins.

The two main arteries and main veins in the circulatory system are:

- The pulmonary artery: carries carbon dioxide-rich blood *from* the heart to the lungs
- The aorta: carries blood *from* the heart to other parts of the body
- The pulmonary veins: bring oxygen-rich blood from the lungs *to* the heart
- The vena cava: brings blood from other parts of the body *to* the heart.

From the heart the large arteries spread out into the body, branching into smaller and smaller arteries and dividing further to form the very small arterioles which in turn lead to the capillaries which are the smallest blood vessels. Capillaries form networks inside all the organs of the body.

The capillaries reunite to form venules (the smallest veins) which join together to form larger veins, which in turn eventually join the major veins that drain into the heart. The arteries and veins are joined through the capillaries to create a circuit that flows through the heart.

Arteries These are tubular structures that carry blood away from the heart. They have thick walls composed of five layers of tissue:

- Inner endothelial coat
- Yellow elastic fibrous coat
- White smooth muscle coat
- Yellow elastic fibrous coat
- Loose connective tissue coat.

Arteries require this thick wall because the blood that they help to pump around the body is under pressure. The elastic tissue is important in maintaining this pressure while the smooth muscle layer controls the size of the artery. This in turn controls the amount of blood flowing through the vessels and the distribution of that blood throughout the body.

Tissues and organs require different amounts of blood at different times. For example, when you are running, your leg muscles require extra blood to supply the energy to work your muscles quickly. After a heavy meal, the digestive system requires extra blood to carry out the digestion of the meal. During pregnancy the foetus requires blood for growth.

If much blood is lost from the body due to injury, the blood pressure is reduced, resulting in a state of shock.

Veins These are also tubular structures but they are larger than the arteries and have thinner walls. They serve to carry blood from the organs of the body back to the heart. The walls of veins have only a small amount of muscle. Inside the veins are a number of valves, scattered along their length at irregular intervals. These valves are necessary to 'push' the blood towards the heart because the pressure of blood within the veins is very low, and the thin, poorly muscled walls cannot pump the blood along.

Capillaries These are very small, thread-like tubes made of endothelial tissue (similar to the inner layer of the arterial walls), a very thin wall which acts as a semi-permeable membrane. This wall allows nutrients, water and oxygen to pass out of the capillary into the surrounding tissues and carbon dioxide and waste products to pass into it.

The heart

The heart is a cone-shaped, hollow, muscular organ situated in the centre of the thorax or chest cavity. It is partly surrounded by a membrane called the pericardium which produces a fluid that acts to lubricate the outside of the heart, which moves constantly as it beats.

The walls of the heart are called the myocardium (meaning 'around the heart' in Greek). The myocardium is made up of a specialised striated involuntary muscle called the cardiac muscle (see page 10).

The heart is divided down the middle by a layer of cardiac muscle called the septum. In the normal healthy human there is no contact between the two sides—blood cannot flow from the left to the right side of the heart.

Each side is further divided into two chambers, an upper chamber called the atrium and a lower chamber called the ventricle. Thus at the top of the heart there are the left and right atrium and at the bottom of the heart are the left and right ventricle.

Between the atrium and ventricle on each side there is a valve called the atrio-ventricular valve (simply referred to as the A-V valve). The A-V valve is made of muscle and controls the flow of blood from one chamber to the other.

Four main vessels carry blood away from and back into the heart. Each vessel leading from the ventricles has a valve called a semi-lunar valve which prevents the blood running back into the heart.

- The pulmonary artery carries blood from the right ventricle to the lungs
- The aorta carries blood from the left ventricle to other parts of the body
- The pulmonary veins bring blood from the lungs to the left atrium
- The vena cava brings blood from other parts of the body to the right atrium.

The 'beating' of the heart is simply the contracting and relaxing of the heart wall. The heart is able to function quite independently of any outside control because it is controlled by impulses sent out by two centres of specialised cardiac cells, the sino-atrial node which governs contraction of the atrium, and the atrio-ventricular node which governs the ventricles. Both these nodes are situated in the muscular heart wall.

Physiology of the circulatory system

The sequence of events that occurs during one complete heartbeat may be summarised thus:

1. Blood enters at the right atrium from the vena cava. At the same time, blood enters the left atrium from the pulmonary vein which comes from the lungs.
2. When both are full of blood, the left and right atrium contract together. This contraction is called the atrial systole.
3. This contraction builds up pressure, forcing open the atrio-ventricular (A-V) valves. Blood is now able to flow into the ventricles which are relaxed.
4. Both atria start to relax, an action known as atrial diastole. At the same time, both ventricles begin contracting (ventricular systole).
5. Pressure in the ventricles increases, causing the A-V valves to snap shut and close off the gap between the atrium and the ventricle.
6. As the pressure continues to rise in the ventricles, the semi-lunar valves open and blood is forced out of both ventricles. The right ventricle pumps blood into the pulmonary artery and the left ventricle pumps the blood into the aorta.
7. The ventricles begin to relax (ventricular diastole) and the semi-lunar valves snap shut. The whole cycle then repeats itself.

These contractions and relaxations (or heartbeats) are controlled by the sino-atrial and atrio-ventricular nodes situated in the wall of the heart.

The efficient working of the circulatory system depends on pressure being maintained, once blood has been forced into the large arteries, by:

- The closure of the semi-lunar valves to prevent the back flow of blood into the heart
- The elasticity of the walls of the arteries. During systole the walls expand to accommodate the extra volume of blood. During diastole the walls recoil, thus maintaining the pressure on the blood inside the artery.

Rate of heartbeat (pulse rate)

Although the heart beats continuously on its own, the nervous system does have some control over the rate of heartbeat and the strength of the contractions. During increased muscular activity, such as running, the amount of blood returned to the heart increases. This causes the pressure in the heart and arteries to rise. In a reflex response, the rate of heartbeat increases. When the pressure in the heart and arteries drops sufficiently, the heartbeat will decrease, again by a reflex action.

Circulatory networks

Four sub-systems of networks make up the circulatory system. Individually they serve particular purposes:

1. *Pulmonary (lung) circulation* This network allows for blood to be recirculated via the lungs so that it can be enriched with oxygen.
2. *Systemic system* This network allows blood to take nutrients to the cells and to remove waste products from the cells.
3. *Hepatic portal system* This directs blood from the spleen, intestines, pancreas and stomach towards the liver, where nutrients are exchanged (e.g. glycogen) while harmful substances are removed.
4. *Lymphatic system* This system removes excess fluid from the cells, originally taken to the cells by the blood.

CHAPTER 2

EQUIPMENT AND FACILITIES

Before commencing regular exercise, you must decide where to exercise, and what equipment or other facilities are needed. This may involve choosing a gymnasium or exercise class to join; but how is the best choice made? If the plan is to exercise at home, decisions must be made about what equipment to purchase, and where at home to exercise.

This chapter is designed to develop an understanding of equipment and facilities, so that more informed choices can be made about these and similar questions.

Aerobic activities can be performed both indoors, e.g. at a gym or in a hall, and outdoors. The type of facilities required will depend on the specific activities being undertaken. Most people consider aerobic exercise to be the typical structured aerobics class or session held in a gym or hall, but aerobic exercise can involve a wide range of other activities such as bike riding, running or swimming, each of which has its own specific equipment requirements. To list all of these is beyond the scope of this book. This chapter will concentrate on the equipment requirements for the structured aerobic class, and include some ideas on selecting equipment for aerobic activities in general.

Pros and cons of indoor exercise
Pros
- Protection against the elements (rain, wind, sun)
- Air temperature can be more readily controlled
- There are usually fewer distractions (vehicles passing by, animals, other people)
- Privacy and personal safety can be more readily maintained.

Cons
- Participants may feel restricted or enclosed.
- There may be less room to move
- The noise from an exercise-to-music class can be annoying to others in the gym, residents living nearby, or people working nearby.

Pros and cons of outdoor exercise
Pros
- Pleasure of exercising in fresh air
- The greater variety of things to observe can reduce boredom.

Cons
- Sun protection is needed
- Wind, rain and glare can be a problem
- Other people watching can discourage proper participation by anyone who is self-conscious
- External noises will make hearing the instructor harder; the instructor also needs to maximise the use of their voice, because the louder the outside environment the more strain is put on the instructor
- Increased level of distractions.

INDOOR FACILITIES

The comfort and fitness benefit derived from exercising indoors can be affected by a number of variables.

Floor conditions
Aerobics classes are best run on a sprung floor to absorb impact. A hard floor will soon cause injuries to both instructor and participants. A

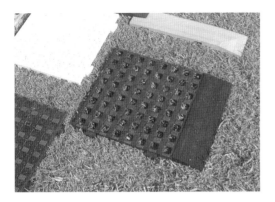

Rubber matting: resilient surfaces such as these are preferable if you are doing exercises which may create an impact problem.

concrete slab floor, even covered with carpet, will always be harder than a timber floor laid over supporting stumps and joists.

The floor surface should be smooth and level, with no uneven boards, cracks or splinters, and should not be too slippery. Ideally a non-slip coating would be applied, which should be checked regularly and re-applied when necessary. Floor coverings are commonly used, but avoid those that might be abrasive, cause itchiness or friction burns, such as some carpet materials, particularly synthetics.

A carpeted floor should have an underlay of a quality appropriate for exercising on. Some underlays are thicker and denser than others, being specially designed to take the heavy wear that they will get from exercise.

Room height
The exercise space should be high enough that no-one will hit their arms on the ceiling when jumping up, nor on any fittings hanging from above (light fittings, fans).

Mirrors
These can be fixed to the walls to allow participants to observe their form and technique. Mirrors also increase the level of safety by allowing participants to be aware of others close by, thereby decreasing the chances of collision. Additionally, instructors facing a mirror can see the class behind them while instructing new

moves and thus be aware if the class is having difficulty following.

Lighting
The level of lighting should allow for good visibility in all parts of the room, but should not be so bright that it causes discomfort.

Air temperature and quality
In summer, air conditioning may be necessary to reduce the likelihood of heat exhaustion. Air conditioners should be regularly serviced to reduce the likelihood of pathogens (e.g. respiratory diseases) breeding in the system.

Access to fresh air can be important, particularly in small rooms or crowded places. If a large group exercises vigorously in a relatively small air-conditioned room, oxygen levels can drop to a point which affects performance and comfort, when an external source of fresh air may be important.

If suitable cooling is not available, good ventilation via open doorways or windows may be sufficient, although this can allow noise and visual distractions from outside to impact on the class. Flyscreens are recommended on open doors or windows to minimise problems from annoying insects.

Entry and exit
In commercial situations, these should be separate and readily accessible. Workplace Health and Safety regulations may vary from State to State. It can also be very annoying (and potentially unsafe) if participants from a class that has just finished are trying to leave by the same door as those who are going to do the next class are trying to get in. If there were to be a fire, or some other emergency, having two or more access points would be very important.

Obstructions
Remove any extraneous items such as pot plants and seating not needed for the exercise program. The fewer items there are in the room/hall, the fewer things there are for participants to trip over or bump into, and the fewer things that require maintenance.

Sound

In commercial situations acoustics should be good, so that participants can clearly and easily hear each other, the instructor, music or a television, where relevant. Avoid using spaces in otherwise empty buildings which echo.

microphone, good stereo system and speakers will generally be necessary, particularly for large classes, and especially where the instructor doesn't have a loud voice or if there is a lot of noise from outside the class. Ideally microphones should be used wherever possible, fixed to the instructor's clothing or a headpiece so that hands are free to demonstrate moves. Clients who find it hard to hear the instructor will tend not to move in the same direction as the rest of the class, which can cause injuries. Music which is too soft, too loud or distorted can reduce motivation and be distracting for all involved.

Steps and other equipment

All equipment must be kept clean and in good condition. Equipment allowed to fall into disrepair, becoming loose, tattered or slippery, or starting to fall apart, increases the risk of injury litigation (i.e. under public liability and professional indemnity).

Stage

Where an instructor demonstrates the exercises from a raised stage or platform, participants can see better, reducing the likelihood of confusion. A stage, however, can create a problem for the instructor due to the risk of falling off. Any raised area should be of a suitable size for the activities being performed, and positioned where all of the class can clearly see it, and where it doesn't create an obstacle when the class members are moving about.

Exercise mats or padding

Exercise mats are often used for floor exercises, increasing comfort and safety and decreasing the risk of back problems. They may be provided by gym management or sometimes by the class participants themselves.

Storage

A suitable 'locker room' area or perhaps shelving should be provided where participants can place bags, towels, jackets, shoes, etc. so that they won't pose a hazard (e.g. tripped over), and can be clearly seen, thus minimising the risk of theft. A nearby safe, secure storage area is required to store any equipment (e.g. mats, steps) regularly used in the aerobics classes.

OUTDOOR AREAS

The comfort and fitness benefit derived from exercising outdoors is also affected by a number of factors.

The surface should be as level as possible (no slope, no uneven areas). It should have a good grip and, depending on the type of activity it is used for, should probably have some resilience to reduce impact.

Any outdoor site must have very good drainage to prevent any water build-up, both on the surface and beneath the surface, causing it to become boggy or soft.

Shelter

Any outdoor area should have as much protection as possible from the elements—windbreaks, shade, shelter from rain.

Distractions

The site should ideally offer minimal visual and auditory distractions to both participants and other people nearby. The most appropriate situation is away from the general public. For example, holding an aerobics class in the park on a Wednesday afternoon would be fine, but not if it interfered with the local Senior Citizens barbecue.

Light and shade

Dappled shade from a canopy of trees can be used as protection from the glare of the sun, but heavy shade on a dull day can make it difficult for some people to follow an instructor's movements. The instructor needs to be aware of sun direction—participants should not look into the sun. Suitable lighting will be needed in an area used for night classes.

Amenities

A suitable place, secure and readily accessed, where participants can place bags and towels, is important. Toilet facilities are also valuable.

Surface

Options for outdoor surfaces include grass/lawn, hard surfaces such as concrete/asphalt/pavers/etc., wooden decks and artificial turf (e.g. Astro-turf). When deciding if a particular outdoor surface is suitable, consider the following:

- Will participants need to sit or lie down to carry out any exercises?
- What is the likely impact on feet and legs?
- Does the surface provide good grip, too much grip for certain exercises, is it too slippery for some exercises, etc.? Does the grip of the surface change if the surface is wet?
- What are the temperature attributes of the surface? Concrete is cold in winter, for example, asphalt is hot in summer, while timber seems to be neutral and generally acceptable. Some artificial surfaces get very hot and may require watering to cool them down.
- The likely degree of sun reflection off the surface (concrete has a high reflective factor and can cause eyestrain, for example).
- The possibility of injury if participants fall or slip (breaks, sprains, skin abrasions).

SURFACES INSIDE AND OUT

A good surface, whether indoors or outside, should exhibit:

- **A good ratio of rebound resilience** Person–surface resilience ratio is a measure of the energy returned after an impact; a low-resilience surface will absorb more of the energy in an impact. Too low a level may be tiring for an aerobic work-out, whereas working

out on a surface with too high a level of resilience would be like exercising on a trampoline.
- **Stiffness** This quality is important if a participant falls. The softer the surface, the less chance of injury. A very soft surface will make the aerobic activity harder to perform (more calories will be burnt), but may not offer good foot support. A very hard surface is more likely to cause injury.
- **Friction** A good level of person–surface friction is important to ensure traction through various exercises and to prevent accidental slipping. Too high a level of friction will restrict foot movement.

All surfaces, whether indoors or out, will over time exhibit wear and tear. This may lead to an increasing possibility of injury as the surface deteriorates. Regular inspection of the surfaces being used is necessary to detect early signs of any problems, so that repair or maintenance can be carried out.

CLOTHING AND FOOTWEAR

Choice of clothing and footwear can aid or hinder movement in aerobic and most other forms of exercise. The most important thing about clothing for aerobic activities is that it is comfortable.

Clothing should be selected in terms of:

- The protection it offers from injury and the sun.
- Light conditions (bright or dull).
- Does it absorb moisture, or resist water absorption? What you choose will depend on what type of activity you are doing; for example, moisture absorption can be important when you are sweating a great deal, while water-resistant jackets can be important for canoeing or whitewater rafting.
- Does it allow suitable freedom of movement?
- Does it give suitable levels of support where required?

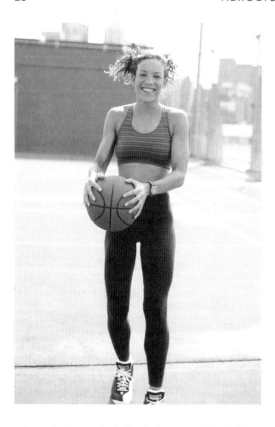

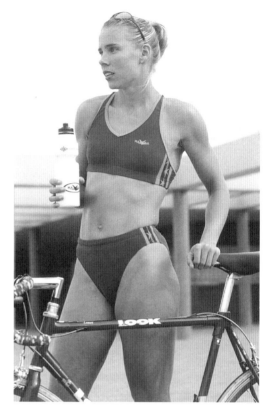

When playing basketball select appropriate clothing to keep body active. Model: Iona Wynter, Jamaican triathlete.

PHOTO: COURTESY RUNNING BARE ACTIVE WEAR

Nici Andronicus modelling suitable clothing for females riding bikes for exercise or in triathlon competition.

PHOTO: COURTESY RIVAL SWIM/TRIATHLON WEAR

- Is it durable? Will it stand up to the rigours of hard exercise? Does it stretch?
- Is it comfortable to wear? Does it bunch or ride up, does it rub?
- Does it have the right appearance for the activity you are carrying out (i.e. is it aesthetically suitable)? This is often dictated by current fashion trends.

TYPES OF FABRIC

Most fitness clothing is constructed from knitted fabrics which permit stretching. Knitted weaves tend to ladder, similar to the way stockings and tights run.

The most popular form of clothing for anyone participating in fitness is anything that is comfortable, warm in cold weather or cool in the heat, and which offers protection from the wind. The sun protection factor is an important consideration for clothing used outdoors, with many manufacturers stating SPF ratings on labelling. In competitive sports the most significant textile products are Elastane and Spandex. Du Pont's Lycra is a superior quality form of Spandex which is blended with other fibres including wool, cotton, rayon and linen to produce various garments suitable for most sports. These Spandex-related products are most popular in aerobic sports such as swimming, cycling and aerobics.

Clothing for other sports such as soccer tends to be made with nylon or polyester. Nylon has traditionally not been particularly

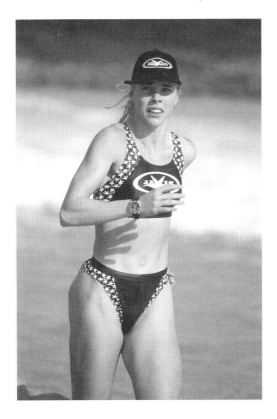

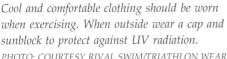

Cool and comfortable clothing should be worn when exercising. When outside wear a cap and sunblock to protect against UV radiation.
PHOTO: COURTESY RIVAL SWIM/TRIATHLON WEAR

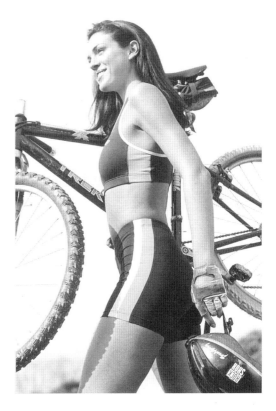

Sportswear made from Tactel™, a high-tech durable fabric designed to carry moisture away from the skin.
PHOTO: COURTESY RUNNING BARE ACTIVE WEAR

popular in many sports as it is considered not to breathe, it clings to the body, and is generally hot and non-flexible in character. New weaving patterns now permit better breathing. Nylon exhibits low staining levels from grass.

Polyester is popular due to its toughness and resilience; it has good memory (it stretches well and returns to the same shape repeatedly), retains its colour and is one of the few textiles that permits sublimation (printing on the material). It is available in weights ranging from super-light-weight to super-heavyweight. Another popular form of polyester is the cloth with holes through-out, sometimes called athletic mesh—it stretches both ways, allows for excellent breathing, but must be dried in the shade.

Footballers tend to prefer traditional fabrics

of cotton/polyester blends for strength, or 100 per cent cotton.

Water-based sports such as rafting require clothing of water-tolerant fabric (e.g. Lycra) and also waterproof clothing where it is important the body remains dry.

FOOTWEAR

Suitable footwear for aerobic activity will depend on:

- The activity to be performed
- The surface on which it is to be performed
- The individual features of a person's foot (i.e. flat, neutral or high-arched).

Cushioning verses stability There is usually a

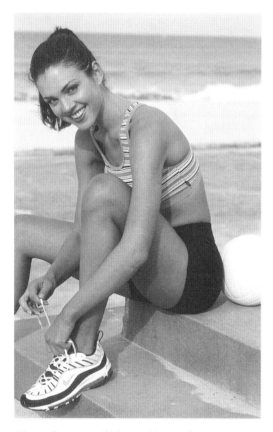

Choose footwear which provides good support during exercise.
PHOTO: COURTESY RUNNING BARE ACTIVE WEAR

trade-off between these two features. A shoe with good cushioning will lose some degree of stability.

Pronation problems Many shoes these days are constructed to take into account the problem where the foot tends to roll inwards. About 25 per cent of people are believed to have this condition, which effectively gives a poor take-off platform, transfers energy inefficiently and increases the risk of injury. Look for shoes with good motion control.

Some feet are not flexible enough to absorb a stress load and so need shoes with good shock-absorbing qualities rather than motion control.

Flexibility Shoes themselves need some degree of flexibility—too much or too little can

reduce the wearer's ability to carry out particular activities or exercises.

Achilles notch This is a small notch in the upper rear ankle tab that contours the back of the shoe to the ankle and Achilles tendon, offering better comfort.

Soles Different materials and patterning provide different degrees of grip, which can change over time as the shoe wears.

Purpose Shoe manufacturers tend to produce shoes specifically for different activities, such as running, weight lifting, aerobics or circuit training. Some make cross-trainers which reputedly are suitable for a range of exercise routines. Each person needs to make up their own mind as to what suits their specific need.

In general, footwear should be well-fitting, provide suitable ankle support and suitable grip. If you are not sure what kind of shoe to use, ask an instructor or gym management for advice. Some gyms and recreation facilities don't allow the use of black-soled footwear, which can leave marks on the floor.

Shoes wear quickly; the sole will lose grip and the internal cushioning break down more quickly the more often the shoe is used. Continuing to use shoes after their support structure and soles have worn increases the risk of injury to feet, ankles, shins, knees and lower back. It is essential that footwear be replaced when necessary. Regular aerobic participants and instructors may need to purchase new shoes as often as every two months.

MUSIC

Music is one of the best ways of stimulating people while they exercise. People may attend or quit exercises class primarily because they like or dislike the music being used.

If you exercise to music at home, choose music which motivates you to exercise and helps you keep an appropriate beat; this might not always be your favourite recording.

In a class situation, an instructor who uses music tapes from ten years ago, or the same tape week after week, risks boring the participants. The presence in the market of music companies set up specifically to provide aerobic tapes for instructors means boredom should never be a problem. Fitness leaders should look to purchasing new tapes as often as every eight weeks.

In an aerobics class where routines and choreography are important, music plays a big role. It needs to be 'bridge-free', meaning all counts are in groups of 8 and 32. Eight counts are referred to as a 'phrase' and 32 counts are known as a 'block'. Music which can be heard in counts of 6, 14 or 27 is almost impossible to use. Using music with 32 counts throughout will allow the leader to count '4, 3, 2 and 1' to introduce the next move. If cueing (counting) is not used, the chance of collisions and injuries amongst class members increases.

Fitness music companies make tapes using music of the correct speed, which is vital for the safety of class. If a fast tape (155 beats per minute) was used for a Step Reebok class, participants would be going mad trying to get up and down on the step—this speed does not give time to perform the movement correctly and is a recipe for disaster. Similarly, using a tape with a Step Reebok speed (124 beats per minute) for a high-impact/advanced class would be slow and boring and would not provide the participants with a challenge.

What each instructor and class likes differs. A 10.30 am female-predominant, low-impact aerobics class might not be willing to jump around to techno or rave music, while the 5.30 pm teenager class would enjoy it. It is important that instructors like the music they are using, but it is more important that their classes like what they hear. One hour of poor quality music of unsuitable style can decrease class numbers.

When you order music from companies which specifically design tapes for fitness classes, you must be certain that the music they have copied is legally licensed. Companies have to pay royalties to governing bodies like ARIA (the Australian Record Industry Association) and AMCOS (the Australasian Mechanical Copyright Owners Society) for the rights to use each piece of music. Taping your own music from a CD and using it in the class is illegal unless you have paid for the rights with AMCOS. This also applies if you copy a tape from another instructor. Illegal copying can cost the gym and the instructor a very hefty fine (up to $10 000) or up to one year's imprisonment.

For details on AMCOS see below. Nightclubs, shops and boutiques have to also pay for the rights to use music. This is done through APRA (the Australian Performing Rights Association).

AMCOS
6–12 Atchinson Street, St Leonards, NSW 2065
Locked Bag 3456, St Leonards, NSW 2065
Phone: (02) 9935 7700
e-mail: info@amcos.com.au

Those people lucky enough to work in an environment with a modern sound system could utilise the pitch-control button, which allows music to be slowed down or speeded up according to the ability of the class or the individual exerciser at home. Slowing down the music for a beginners' class struggling to cope with the speed and the coordination of the movements is often a good move.

Maintaining the system in good condition is an important aspect of keeping management costs down. If instructors are careless and care little for the equipment, a gym could be buying a new sound system or parts (tape-deck door and buttons) every year or so. The tape-decks need to be cleaned out regularly and the heads checked to prevent tapes being damaged. New tapes may have to be purchased more frequently if the music system is not kept in good condition. Who is responsible—the management or the instructor for not cleaning the tape-deck heads, or the instructor for not reminding management?

CHARACTERISTICS OF EQUIPMENT

A wide range of equipment for aerobic exercise is available. Often the advertising for such machines enthusiastically promises a fantastic all-round work-out. In reality, the benefits derived from using aerobic equipment can usually be derived just as well through exercises which require no equipment at all. There are, however, some advantages to using aerobic equipment, not the least being the convenience of exercising in a relatively confined space, and in a pleasant environment.

In general, less equipment is used for structured aerobic classes than for many other gymnasium-based activities.

When choosing a piece of equipment, whether a bike, treadmill, rower or something else, you should always consider the following:

Functionality Does it do what you bought it for? Does it do other things? How effectively does it do each thing/function/task?

Safety Is it safe to operate/use? Is it safe to others? Is it safe to repair/service?

Cost This includes initial, operating and maintenance costs.

Durability How hard-wearing is it?

Longevity How long will it last?

Maintenance How often is maintenance required and how easy is it to do?

Aesthetics Does the appearance suit the place where it is to be used (e.g. gym equipment)?

Availability of parts Are parts readily available? Do they need to be ordered in, or even imported from overseas?

Technical expertise required Do you have the expertise to use the equipment? Can you readily be trained in its use?

Warranty Does the equipment have a warranty? How long is it for (e.g. lifetime or a few years)? What does the warranty cover? Can you purchase an extended warranty, and would such a warranty be cost-effective?

Note: Figures quoted for energy consumption using the following pieces of equipment should be used as a guide only. Energy consumption will vary according to such things as the efficiency of the equipment being used, the speed at which the activity is being carried out, and the conditions under which the activity is being carried out (e.g. riding a bike over smooth or rough terrain).

BIKES

There are two main types of bikes; stationary (used inside, normally in a gymnasium), and mobile (used outside).

A 60-minute work-out on a stationary cycle with levers can burn 509–709 calories; on a stationary cycle without levers, 498–604 calories.

The Australian Compliance Standard for exercise (stationary) bikes (AS4092) states that bikes must have no protruding sharp parts on which people may be injured, and that the wheels and other moving parts must be fully

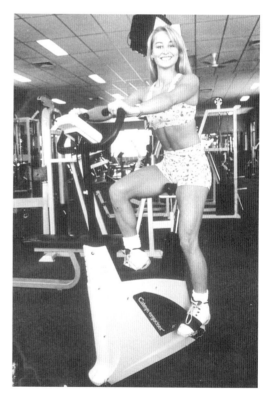

In a well-stocked gym, bikes are a popular activity. Model: Kerryn Cormick (Miss Fitness Victoria 1999).

enclosed to prevent the possibility of injury. International and Australian manufacturing standards for the protection of purchasers and users are extensively used in Australia as a benchmark for manufacturing quality.

All gym equipment should be produced by an accredited ISO9001/AS3901 manufacturer. All legitimate ISO9001/AS3901 accredited manufacturers can provide:

- The name of the certifying accreditation authority, e.g. Standards Australia, SGS International Certification Services PL
- A file reference number of the manufacturer's accreditation. This should be asked for when receiving quotations for equipment. This is an internationally recognised standard for quality in design and workmanship.

Mobile bikes

There are many different types of mobile bikes, designed with different features to suit different purposes. For example:

- Road bikes
- Touring bikes: used for long distances, and have dropped handlebars
- Racing bikes: designed for speed, are light, thin and aerodynamic
- Sport bikes: have features of both road and touring bikes, and are best for longer rides (perhaps 15 km or so), or more where speed is used
- Mountain or all-terrain bikes: have an upright sitting position, sturdy construction, good-grip tyres, straight handlebars
- Hybrids: a blend of road and mountain bike, lighter than a mountain bike, but not as fast as a road bike; straight handlebars, good for commuting, running errands and short distances.

Stationary bikes

These can range from the basic home unit to the state-of-the-art electronically programmed commercial models. They are a very useful and popular piece of gym equipment.

All exercise bikes need to be user-friendly, with a basic manual program which is activated simply by pedalling. To change to a different program the bike should have clear instructions on its use and push-button operation.

A bike must be comfortable, with adjustable seat and frame so that the bike can be adjusted to the correct biomechanical set-up for each user. Pedal straps should be quick-release and adjustable for safety and comfort. Heart-rate monitors, including Polar™ chest strap or ear clip, are useful additions to any exercise bike, giving the user feedback and helping to motivate increased effort. Some heart-rate monitors include safety shut-off features that react to the user's heart-rate exceeding the specified heart-rate to age data programmed into them beforehand.

The recumbent cycle provides a unique alternative, especially for the poorly conditioned, pregnant or rehabilitating user. With a wider seat and lower back support it is more comfortable than standard exercise bikes. Other benefits include increased work-out for the buttocks and back of the thigh because of the seating angle. The recumbent cycle is easier on the heart and allows higher calorie burn-off for less heart effort; it also allows the user to watch TV or a video or even to read. This style of exercise bike is becoming more and more popular in gyms.

It is possible to incorporate some resistance exercises in with use of the recumbent bike by using dumbbells or specially designed pulley machines. This way both an aerobic and a resistance work-out can be done at the same time.

Selecting a bike, either mobile or stationary

- Consult with specialist bike suppliers to determine which type of bike (and associated equipment) best suits your needs (and price range).
- Choose the right type according to the expected use, for example, a road bike is faster than a mountain bike, but it can be readily damaged by rough road edges and unmade roads.
- Check for the right size and comfort:

  1. Height—straddle the bike and measure the distance between the bike's top bar

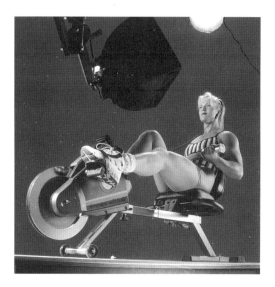

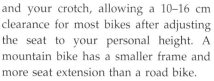

Recumbent cycle ergometer with ear attachment heart monitor.
PHOTO: COURTESY ONLY FITNESS (AUST.) PTY LTD

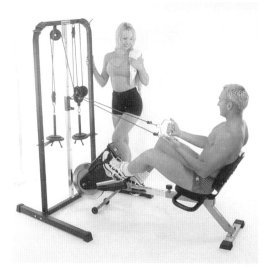

Powerobics system: This combines a pulley weights system with a recumbent cycle to allow a larger number of muscle groups to be worked at the same time.
PHOTO: COURTESY ONLY FITNESS (AUST.) PTY LTD

and your crotch, allowing a 10–16 cm clearance for most bikes after adjusting the seat to your personal height. A mountain bike has a smaller frame and more seat extension than a road bike.

2. Seat and handlebar adjustment—handlebars should be the same height as the seat or about 3 cm lower. The seat should be positioned so that the lower leg is at a 25–30 degree angle from the vertical when the ball of the foot is resting on the pedal at its lowest point.

- Frames can be made of a variety of materials; if the bike is to take more wear and tear than the 'average' recreational bike (e.g. a mountain bike) then you need a stronger frame than usual. High tensile steel frames are common. Both chromium-molybdenum (Cr-Mo) and alloy frames are lighter and stronger, but a lot more expensive, and are best suited to those with plenty of money to spare, and/or for competition where weight is important.

- Wheels which are made of lighter materials (e.g. alloy rims) will make a bike much more responsive, but as with frames choose a metal that will suit the use (road, off-road). Quick-release hubs are an advantage in competition bikes where time is of the essence.

- Older-style bikes use cotter pins on the cranks, but these wear and can come loose with heavy use, so cotterless cranks are preferable.

- Test ride any bike you might be considering purchasing to assess its comfort level.

- When selecting a recumbent bike check it out for comfort and the type of wheel resistance mechanism (whether magnetic or strap.)

Additional equipment

On-road and off-road riders should consider buying:

- Helmet (essential)
- Goggles
- Pump
- Repair kit
- Pressure gauge
- Seat pack

- Water bottle
- Lock.

Heart monitors are beneficial but not essential.

In the indoor gym, the only additional equipment required is a drink bottle and a towel.

Indoors and outdoors, you need comfortable, appropriate clothing.

Using a stationary bike

Posture: Maintain straight back.
Grip: Hold the handlebars firmly—do not grasp tightly.
Feet: Wear good supportive shoes, and use straps for the feet if they are there.
Shoulders: Do not hunch shoulder forwards.
Seat: Adjust the seat so that the knees are slightly bent when the pedal is at lowest point.

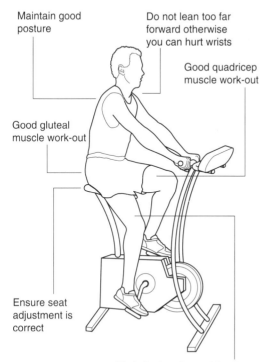

Maintain good posture

Do not lean too far forward otherwise you can hurt wrists

Good quadricep muscle work-out

Good gluteal muscle work-out

Ensure seat adjustment is correct

Work the legs by pushing down with one leg and pulling up with the other. The foot strap permits the upward pull motion

Spinning

Spinning is a fitness system that uses stationary bikes to simulate real road riding by altering the positions of handles and seats and the degree of 'road-resistance' on a flywheel.

Spinning can burn up to 500 calories in a 40-minute ride session.

Riders are best off wearing a heart monitor to measure heart-rate throughout the work-out; they should be aware of maximum efficiency and safe workload limits.

Instructors motivate participants by using imagery. For example, riders may be asked to reduce the cycle's resistance and picture themselves riding along the beach. The instructor can describe the seagulls, lapping waves, sun and bathers, to mentally relax the riders so that they enjoy the exercise session and divert their minds from the physical exercise they are undertaking. Music is frequently used to enhance emotion and speed up or slow down the exercise intensity.

STEPPING OR STAIR-CLIMBING MACHINES

These are machines which simulate the actions of climbing or stepping. They are used primarily for cardiovascular conditioning, but can also be used for weight loss and conditioning the calves, thighs and buttocks.

A 60-minute work-out on a stair machine can burn 637–746 calories. Less expensive steppers (usually intended for home use) are not motorised, and offer fewer options. A decent stepper will offer variety in its resistance and pace, ideally with climbing modes of steeper ascent and increased pace for the better-conditioned user. You will be able to choose to step fast or slow, to take high or low steps, and to push against a greater or lesser force.

By mixing stepping with other aerobic activities, a person can spread the work being done in an aerobic work-out across a greater range of muscles. The benefit of adding exercise variety is a major argument for incorporating stepping into an aerobic work-out where the option to use such a machine is available.

Machines can either be dependent-action in type, where the steps or pedals are joined together with a belt or cable, or independent-action, where they are not connected. On a dependent machine, the left step comes up when the right is pushed down, and vice versa. Independent machines stop the user from shifting their weight from side to side—something which tends to happen when using a dependent machine. This side-to-side shifting of weight can reduce the effectiveness of the exercise. Independent-action machines are considered safer and their use is less likely to result in injury.

The three main types of stepping machine are: hydraulic cylinder, air resistance, and mechanised computer-controlled.

- **Hydraulic cylinder machines** use air or hydraulic fluid inside a cylinder to provide resistance. Less sophisticated models offer only one level of resistance, more expensive ones allow resistance to be increased as the user's fitness increases. Independent-action types place a greater stress on the cylinder, so a heavier duty, more durable cylinder is needed. Generally, the thicker the diameter of the cylinder, the stronger it will be.
- **Air resistance machines** use a fan to provide the resistance. As the stepping rate increases or decreases, the fan speed increases or decreases, changing the resistance accordingly. These machines are generally more expensive and more durable than the cylinder type. Some models also incorporate a resistance belt as a further means of controlling the workload.
- **Mechanised computer-controlled machines** control resistance by a brake which in turn is controlled by a computer. These machines are the most expensive type, but also the most controllable. Resistance can be varied across a pre-set time period, controlled by a computer program, to provide a sequence of varying workloads. In addition, because the workload is computer-controlled, it is possible to provide accurate feedback on the work being done (e.g. calories used,

duration). A range of different braking mechanisms is found in this type of machine. The cheapest is an 'eddy current' brake, which may only have a short lifespan. Electromagnetic braking is durable and fairly accurate, but may not provide adequate resistance for a heavier person (108 kg or heavier). An alternator braking mechanism is the best, most durable and accurate.

Selecting a stepping machine
- The construction of any stepper, manual or mechanised, should be sturdy.
- The better manual machines will allow resistance to be adjusted to vary the workload.
- The better mechanised machines are relatively expensive but offer greater ease of adjusting to different slopes and pace, and may include extra options such as a heart-rate monitor.
- The handles should be comfortable and adjustable to accommodate people of varying heights.
- A heart-rate monitor may or may not be provided. Some modern machines incorporate heart-rate monitors in their handles.
- In a computer-controlled machine, look for flexibility in the variety of program options offered.
- Where possible, choose an independent-action stepping machine.

Using a stepping machine
Posture: Maintain a straight back with head looking forward and upward, with shoulders back.

Grip: Hold rails/sides lightly—do not grasp tightly.

Arms: Move arms in synchronisation with leg movements as though you were walking up stairs.

Do not lean or crouch forwards as this can increase back strain.

Steppers with moving arms
A variation on the normal stepping machine is one with moving arms designed to add arm

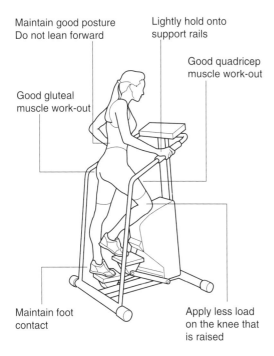

Maintain good posture
Do not lean forward

Lightly hold onto
support rails

Good quadricep
muscle work-out

Good gluteal
muscle work-out

Maintain foot
contact

Apply less load
on the knee that
is raised

movements into a stepping exercise (e.g. the Aerobic X-Press Machine). Standing on two platforms, the feet press up and down, rotating in an ellipse (similar to a stepping machine but an elliptical motion). At the same time, the arms move in opposition to the foot action (i.e. when the left arm moves forward, the left foot moves back; the right foot moves forward and the right arm moves back).

TREADMILLS

Treadmills are used for fat loss and cardiovascular training. They are relatively safe, although some instruction is necessary initially, and comfortable. The better treadmills have a shock-absorbing deck which can reduce impact, compared to jogging on the roads, by one-third. Treadmills can be used for fitness testing, rehabilitation work or the warm-up/cool-down down components of an exercise routine. They can have the flexibility to provide a gentle walk or a heart-pumping run. With some models you can also increase the incline of the treadmill to increase resistance and therefore the intensity of the work-out without needing to increase speed.

A 60-minute work-out on a treadmill can burn around 705–865 calories.

Some types of treadmill can be programmed to provide target maximum heart-rate (MHR) percentages, when used in conjunction with heart-monitor straps.

A treadmill can be used as an alternative to running outdoors when weather conditions are not suitable. You can watch television while exercising. Some of the more expensive models incorporate video displays that simulate changing scenery as you run. Motorised treadmills tend to provide superior aerobic work-outs compared to manual treadmills.

Choosing a treadmill

- A mechanised treadmill is both safer and more useful than a non-mechanised machine on which the speed is not controllable.
- Coated high-alloy steel is better than aluminium. Avoid plastic.
- A welded frame is better than a bolted one.
- Frames should be comfortable and positioned so as not to obstruct movement.
- Preferably select a machine with a continuous-duty horsepower more than 1.5.
- Speed range should be a smooth transition from 0 to 10 or more kph.
- The tread-belt should be long enough to permit comfortable strides, and wide enough to eliminate the fear of stepping off the edge.
- The belt should be strong enough to provide adequate support, but still absorb much of the impact from the user.
- The deck should be strong, should not overheat and should require only minimal maintenance.
- The incline mechanism needs to be both strong (if manual) and smooth (if electronic), and should not move once in position.
- Electronic control panels/gadgets must be reliable and able to be repaired if they break down. You pay more for more gadgets. They should be positioned where the user can readily reach them at all times while exercising.

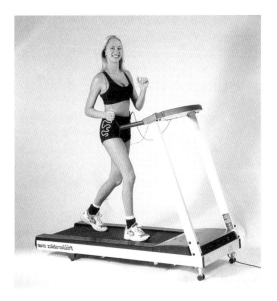 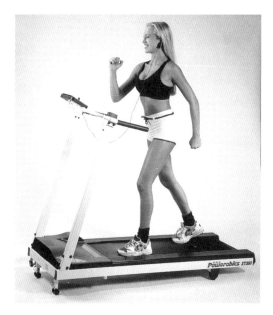

Motorised treadmill with heart monitor which clips onto the ear.
PHOTO: COURTESY ONLY FITNESS (AUST.) PTY LTD

- Heart-rate monitors designed as chest straps are more reliable than ear and finger clips.
- Choose a machine with a quality mat/tread that will not require adjustment or tightening too often.

Using a treadmill

Posture: Maintain an erect stance.

Grip: Keep hands free, using the handles only to regain balance.

Arms: Swinging naturally at the sides.

Do not set the speed of the treadmill to High; start off at a comfortable level and adjust the speed carefully till you reach the desired level of work-out. Don't exercise to the point where you cannot reduce the speed of the treadmill safely without getting off to catch your breath.

Footwear: Good footwear is essential. Don't use a treadmill with bare feet, as the surface can get very hot with prolonged use, and bare feet can blister.

Note: Before you get on the treadmill, make sure the tread has started rolling so its speed is observable. Step with heel-to-toe technique with long, full strides.

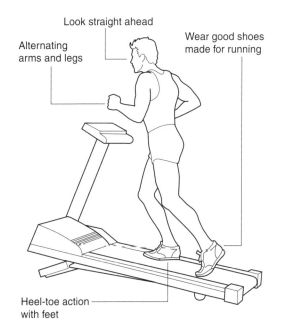

Look straight ahead

Wear good shoes made for running

Alternating arms and legs

Heel-toe action with feet

SKI MACHINES

A ski machine simulates the action of skiing.

The feet are placed on two boards which slide forwards and backwards. The hands grip either handles attached to a pulley system, not unlike some weight machines, or poles (full-length arms) attached to levers.

Many machines, particularly the pulley-system types, also have a padded hip-rest which you can push against with the front of the body (this helps maintain balance). Others depend on the user holding poles to maintain balance.

A 60-minute work-out can burn 600 calories or more.

A ski machine can provide a particularly good aerobic work-out, some would say better than that provided by most other types of aerobic equipment, because it spreads the work-load over more muscle groups than other machines. On a bike or stepping machine, for example, the legs do most of the work; on a ski machine the arms are also given a considerable work-load.

Choosing a ski machine

There are two main types of ski machines; those which have the movements operating independently of each other; and those which have the movements linked (dependent-action types). On the dependent-action machines the 'skis' are linked so that when one slides forward the other automatically slides back. The independent machines are a little more difficult to use at first, but a well-coordinated person should master this type within a few hours. Independent types give a better work-out, but where the user has coordination difficulties the dependent type is probably more suitable.

The cost of machines can vary considerably according to sturdiness of construction and the variables built in. The hip-rest should be adjustable to suit the height of the user. The speed or resistance and slope may also be adjusted. A good machine also offers feedback features such as a heart-rate monitor and a calculation of calories burnt.

It is always wise to try out a machine before buying it. Fifteen minutes of use will usually enable you to effectively gauge the appropriateness of a machine for a particular person's needs.

Using a ski machine

Posture: Lean slightly forward, using the entire torso.

Grip: Maintain a firm but relaxed hand grip.

Arms: Keep elbows low.

Feet: Lift your heel as you push backwards off your foot.

Do not allow feet to pass forward beyond the torso or abdominal support. Do not bend forward at waist.

Note: Position the support pad just below the belly button.

ROWING MACHINES

Rowing machines allow a user to simulate the action of rowing.

They generally consist of a sliding seat, footrests, and a handle or handles attached to a pulley system. The resistance on the pulley system can normally be varied, and a good machine will incorporate a programmable feedback panel (showing calories burnt, distance travelled, etc.) and a range of program sequences of varying intensities.

This type of exercise has the advantage of being low impact, but principally works the upper body, with little leg work being done unless the seat slides along its supporting rails.

A 60-minute work-out can burn 606–739 calories.

Modern rowing machines can be combined with sophisticated computer software and audio-visuals to produce interesting and even exciting challenges for gymnasium users. One program, for example, allows the user to race for the finish line in a challenging regatta—complete with the sounds of a starting gun and cheering crowd. As an added thrill, a shark swims into view and devours part of the competing crew. The user then gets a low-intensity interval before one last push to finish. The user is caught up in the animation of the program and the work-out is more engaging as well as being designed to elicit maximum effort.

Selecting a machine

A good-quality rowing machine will be of sturdy construction, and offer plenty of flexibility in program options. It should be comfortable to use, and the foot straps should be adjustable and hold the feet firm.

As with most equipment, a reasonable guarantee period will provide some indication of good quality.

Using a rowing machine

Posture: Keep a straight back, look straight ahead.
Grip: Grip width should ideally be around the same width as the shoulders.
Arms: Extended out on the pull—pull the bar to the upper chest.
Legs: In front of the body with feet in line with knees. On a machine with a sliding seat the knees bend forwards and backwards with slight flexion in the trunk.
Do not let arms go too far forward in scapular extension, as this can cause back strain.

AIR RIDERS

These machines have an action similar to an old-fashioned rocking horse. The user sits on a seat like a bike seat, with the feet on footrests like bike pedals which don't rotate, and the hands on handlebars like the handlebars of a bike. When the feet are pushed and/or the handlebars pulled, the non-motorised machine moves like a rocking horse.

These machines have become popular recently due to heavy promotion. They are most suited to beginners at the start of an aerobic exercise program. People who are already reasonably fit will obtain little benefit from such machines. They may have more applications among people with limited capabilities, such as the unfit elderly or people recovering from injury.

There is a small degree of abdominal and biceps activity, but the main muscles used tend to be the hamstrings. The height of the user may result in different muscles being exercised. The effort exerted by the arms relative to the legs can be varied in order to work one set of limbs more than the other.

Low back pain has been reported by users of some types of air rider, so care is needed to ensure correct posture is maintained throughout the exercise.

Riders can also be used to provide total body warm-ups before cross-training with other activities.

Selecting an air rider

Always try the machine out first to ensure you like the movement, feel comfortable and safe with the ride, and that resistance changes can be made. Prices and construction do not vary a great deal, but subtle differences in design can make one machine more comfortable than another for a person of a particular body size and shape.

Using an air rider

Posture: Maintain an erect stance.
Grip: Hold handlebars firmly.
Arms: Different muscles can be worked by varying the position and the way the handlebars are gripped, i.e. underhand or overhand.
Legs: Keep feet in shoes with footrest straps in place.
Do not lean forward or back with the movements.

AIR WALKERS

An air walker is basically two rocking footrests suspended from a frame. The user places one foot on each footrest, then moves the legs forwards and backwards as if walking, but without lifting the feet from the footrests.

These machines have been promoted heavily on television and through chain stores.

Research in the USA by the American Council on Exercise (ACE) compared two machines (Airofit and Fitness Flyer). The outcome: long strides burnt more calories than short strides; the machines work the muscles at the hip and the front and back of the thighs. The conclusion: such machines 'are best suited for improving muscular endurance, not strength'; and 'an already fit person will get limited benefit out of these machines'. (For more details of this trial, access the website: http://www.acefitness.org/ and request a copy of *Fitness Matters*, Vol. 3, No. 3.)

Selecting an air walker

Look for long-lasting powdercoated or treated metal. Joints should be welded into position rather than bolted. As most air walkers are purchased boxed and assembled at home, for safety reasons ensure all connections are firm otherwise the machine may fall apart, or parts come loose in mid-stride.

Using an air walker

Posture: Maintain an erect stance.
Grip: Use either a gentle hold on the hand grips, or do not use them at all.
Arms: Moved in relation to the legs in the opposing direction, in the same fluid movement as when walking.
Legs: Move the legs in a smooth striding motion. *Do not* aim to do the splits, i.e. do not extend legs to their full extent in mid-stride as this can overstretch the muscles and may cause more harm than good.

KANGAROO JUMPS/BOOTS

This equipment consists of a pair of boots with a spring attached to each. The spring is made of two strong, arched pieces of plastic, rather like two bananas sitting one on top of the other to make an oval shape. The boot is a strong ski-type boot which provides excellent ankle support, similar to a rollerblade boot. When jumped on, the springs begin to straighten towards each other, according to the weight of the person, then return to normal position, thus providing a bounce. When a heavier person creates a greater force downwards, this causes the spring to react with a greater force up (i.e. there is a natural adjustment to compensate for people of differing weights).

These boots are great fun to use and are becoming increasingly popular in aerobics classes and on the streets. They provide a great alternative to a run or power walk. The spring action works to absorb shock, similar to a kangaroo jumping; they are very good for the joints, and provide a great cardiorespiratory work-out, with emphasis on the thigh and gluteal area. They are very easy to use once the exerciser has got the hang of them, and they can be very popular with the keen rollerblader.

AEROBIC BOUNCER

This is a mini trampoline, circular in shape, usually no larger than 75 cm in diameter. The edge should be covered with padding for safety and the springs also covered to stop the user landing on them.

The aerobic bouncer is popular in circuit classes and for home use. It is safe and easy to use, especially in front of the television to prevent boredom; however, there must be plenty of clear space around the bouncer, and no objects above it (low-hanging light fittings, for example) which could be hit as the exerciser bounces. The bouncer may be difficult to use for long periods on its own because it can become tedious, but is great for providing variety in a class situation. The bouncing motion is not as effective as jogging unless the user is super-energetic.

EQUIPMENT SPECIFIC TO AEROBICS CLASSES
MATS

These provide a comfortable base on which to do floor exercises at the conclusion of a class. They are intended to prevent bruising, abrasions and friction burns. Mats should be durable (both cover and filling) and well-stitched so they don't fall apart easily. The surface should not be too slippery and the filling fairly firm. In other words, the mat should be comfortable, but not so comfortable that the user sinks into it, making it hard to do the exercise or maintain balance. Mats should be small and light enough to be readily moved around and stored.

STEPS

Step classes are a very popular format in aerobics and provides the exerciser with a good cardiovascular and leg work-out. Steps need to be adjustable to cater for individuals of varying heights, lever lengths and ability levels; they must be stable and not rock when people stand on them. The width and length of the stepping surfaces must be sufficient to allow the user to comfortably step up, on and off, and the surface itself strong enough to support repeated impact. The steps should be light enough to be readily carried by users. The base should have a non-slip, protective covering that prevents damage to the floor surface and reduces the likelihood of it slipping in use. The recommended steps are made by Reebok, the creators of this type of activity; many of the imitations are smaller and less stable in structure.

Steps provide a good cardiovascular work-out if performed and instructed correctly. Instructors must be suitably qualified.

STRETCH BANDS

Also called Dyna Bands, this rubber stretch equipment is strong enough to provide a suitable level of resistance, but not so hard to stretch that it becomes too hard. The bands are durable enough to cope with large amounts of repeated stretching. They are used for rehabilitation purposes and for a different type of resistance training within aerobics classes.

POWER BARS

This type of class is a barbell resistance class performed to music. Each body part is worked to one 5-minute track and the weight of the bar can be altered each time. For example, a barbell with weights for a leg track would be different to the one used for a tricep track. This type of class raises the heart-rate and provides a good form of resistance training. It also increases the likelihood of males going into the gym/aerobics room because of the overall body conditioning work-out.

SLIDE REEBOK

This is a different form a cardiovascular work-out where the participant wears special booties over their shoes and slides side to side on a slippery piece of rubber, which is approximately 1.5 metres long and 0.75 metres wide. Safety is extremely important and the instructor needs to know the exact precautions to take to limit risk of injuries. This is a great cardiovascular work-out and excellent for the legs, especially the inner thighs. Slide Reebok is limited in the actions that can be performed; an entire 60-minute class might be boring after the second or third time. It is ideal to use as part of a class for variety.

AEROBIC HOME EQUIPMENT

If you are thinking of setting up a home gym there are a few things that first need to be determined:

* Your (and your family's) present fitness level
* Available funds
* The objective of the exercise (i.e. aerobic or resistance training, or both)
* The space available to perform a range of exercises.

As a guide the following table indicates the approximate area required for different pieces of aerobic equipment. Space should also be provided to allow for clear access to and from each of the separate pieces of equipment you might have.

Treadmill	3 square metres
Bike	1–2 square metres
Stair climber	1–2 square metres
Rowing machine	2 square metres
Ski machine	2–2.5 square metres

Aerobic equipment should be light enough in resistance to permit at least a 20-minute workout with smooth motions.

When thinking of cost, always remember that you get what you pay for. Well-built and reliable equipment will cost more initially, but in the long run will still be in use in years to come. Cheaper brands may have broken down many years earlier. Do your homework to determine what you need to look for in deciding on the best equipment for your needs in your price range. Second-hand equipment is cheaper than new, but be aware that damage, or significant wear and tear, may have occurred, and a guarantee will generally not be available.

When selecting equipment, consider:

- Freedom of movement
- The ease of changing resistance or mode of action
- Easy-to-follow instructions and computer display units
- Sturdy and secure hand-rails and overall construction
- Safety features such as safety switches, stop buttons, guards, limiters to range-of-motion
- Noise of equipment in operation
- Serviceability and warranty.

When making your selections, think about what you like to do. If you are a walker, then invest in a treadmill. If you enjoy snow skiing, then invest in a cross-country skiing machine. If you enjoy bicycle rides, then purchase a stationary cycle.

To ensure you do not waste money by not using the equipment, it is important to set home goals and visualise your desired outcome, whether that is an improved shape or just being more active.

Consider utilising your television or stereo system in conjunction with the equipment to help decrease boredom during exercise.

More adventurous equipment

- 'Computerised sparring partners' provide aerobic exercise and cross-training for boxers and martial arts fans. They consist of

a free-standing punching bag with a built-in computer, which stands on a circular plastic base.

- 'Elliptical fitness cross-trainers' simulate cross-country skiing, stair-climbing, running and cycling. Products like these have been in the gyms for years and are now slowly making their way into homes.
- Step Jet™: a personalised fitness watercraft on which the user pumps the step pads by normal walking motions to generate forward momentum for the watercraft. This piece of equipment can be used as a mode of transport over canals (so the advertisements suggest) or as an alternative to walking the footpaths and jarring the legs.

Maintaining equipment

At all times all equipment should be:

- Kept clean.
- Kept lubricated where appropriate (moving parts), being careful not to leave oil or grease where users may come into contact with it. This can not only create unsafe (slippery) conditions but also stain clothing.
- Regularly checked, and any problems remedied by repair or replacement as soon as possible. If the problem poses a safety risk, the equipment must be taken out of use until it is repaired.
- Kept accurate—this is important where any sort of measuring device is used, such as heart-rate monitors and distance meters.
- Kept in a safe, secure place to reduce theft, vandalism and wrongful use, and also to prevent access by small children.

OUTDOORS OR PARK EQUIPMENT FOR AEROBIC EXERCISE

Fitness trails provide a great opportunity to improve overall health and cardiovascular capacity.

These trails have been constructed in

various towns and cities, usually by Parks departments, for the public to use as a form of fitness activity. Over a distance generally at least of two or three kilometres, a series of stations, usually well posted with instructions, encourage participants to carry out specific exercise routines.

These exercises can incorporate a range of aerobic, resistance and flexibility exercises. Depending on how many of each exercise you do, how quickly you do them, how much rest you have between different sets of exercises, and how fast you get from station to station, the fitness trail session can be orientated towards either a resistance work-out or an aerobic work-out.

Exercise stations can include:

- Monkey bars and chin-up bars
- Hurdles
- Log hops
- Step ups
- Bounce jumps
- Treadmills
- Stomach exercises such as crunches
- Burpies or star jumps
- Running on the spot and, of course,
- Running between the various stations.

OTHER OUTDOOR AEROBIC ACTIVITIES

As an alternative to home or gym aerobics classes, activities that can promote aerobic conditioning and add variety to the average aerobics class include the following:

- Runs in the park
- Outdoor fitness trails in parks
- Beach running
- Shallow beach/river running
- In-line skating, ice-skating
- Rock climbing
- Whitewater rafting/canoeing
- High-rise step running
- Horse riding
- Swimming
- Roller-blading
- Trampolining
- Wrestling or other martial arts
- One-on-one basketball
- Handball
- Squash, tennis, other ball sports.

As with any exercise, the benefits will depend on such things as how long you do the activity, at what intensity, how long you rest between sessions, and what types of equipment you are using.

CHAPTER 3

TYPES OF AEROBIC EXERCISE

There are many more options for aerobic exercise than most people realise!

The obvious things are swimming, jogging, cycling and working out in an aerobics exercise class. Less obvious options include participation in work and other sporting activities—but just as some sports are more appropriate for aerobic conditioning than others, some types of physical work do more for aerobic fitness than others.

This chapter will help you understand how to get the best aerobic fitness benefit from some of these options.

First—How often? How hard?

Before beginning any fitness or exercise program, ensure you obtain a medical clearance.

For any appreciable benefit, you should train at least three times a week.

Your heart-rate should be raised, and maintained at an elevated level for at least 20 minutes each time; to do this with a suitable warm-up and cool-down period requires 30 or 35 minutes at least.

> You need to exercise at least three times a week for around 35 minutes or more each time.

Longer periods of exercise, perhaps up to 50 or 60 minutes, are even better. More frequent exercise, perhaps even daily, can be very beneficial, provided you don't over-stress the body.

Alternate the days on which you do hard and light exercise or training. Excessively hard training on two consecutive days can create excess stress on joints, ligaments and muscles, and deplete muscle glycogen levels. One very hard session each week is adequate. You can train or exercise daily, but be sympathetic to how your body feels and do not persist if pain increases or the legs become very heavy (even if it is only a

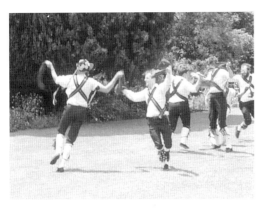

Morris dancing—most types of dancing are good for maintaining aerobic fitness.

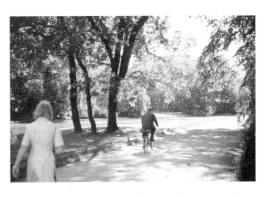

Walking or cycling to and from work is one option for maintaining aerobic fitness that many people should consider.

light day). There is just as much danger in over-training as there is in under-training!

Keeping hydrated

During aerobic exercise it is important to keep hydrated by consuming adequate amounts of water. Water is important for the sportsperson during exercise because it maintains blood volume, regulates heart function and helps maintain normal body temperature. When body temperature increases during exercise, especially in hot conditions encountered during a marathon, for example, the body must reduce this temperature to keep body functions at normal levels. Blood flow to the skin increases with higher temperatures, and heat is transferred out of the body through sweat. This increases fluid loss, thus water is required to top up fluid levels.

Loss of total body fluid

An excessive amount of fluid loss can cause problems for the athlete, summarised here:

- 1–2%: loss of appetite and discomfort
- 3–4%: poor performance, dry mouth, flushed skin and nausea
- 5–6%: reduced ability to regulate own body temperature, poor concentration
- 8%: dizziness, weakness, mental confusion
- 10–11%: heat exhaustion, heatstroke, possible death.

To reduce the risk of these problems occurring, adequate hydration must be maintained. Before exercise a minimum of 2 or 3 glasses of water should be consumed. *Never* wait until you are thirsty because this means you are already dehydrated. Act before thirst sets in. During exercise it is recommended that 120–250 ml of water be taken every 15 minutes. Small volumes should be drunk, as large amounts of fluid actually leave the stomach more quickly than smaller volumes. Once exercise has ceased it is time to replace all lost fluids; this process should begin straight away.

The best fluids to consume during exercise which continues for more than one to one-and-a-half hours are specially formulated sports drinks which supply carbohydrates and some electrolytes (sodium and potassium). The electrolytes help the body absorb fluids faster. Drinks with too high a concentration of carbohydrates or electrolytes will remain in the body for longer, causing discomfort.

After exercise, drinks high in carbohydrates will help replenish stores of energy. Sports drinks, soft drinks or flavoured milk all assist the recovery phase.

EXERCISE MOVEMENT COMPONENTS

Every exercise is composed of a combination of positions which different parts of the body remain in, or move through, over a certain period of time.

Movement can be analysed in terms of the following components:

- Foot placement
- Position of hips (from all directions)
- Angle between hip and upper leg at different stages of the movement
- Angle of the ankle (foot to lower leg) at various stages
- Angle of knee at various stages
- Position of arms
- Angle of back (e.g. at right angles to water surface)
- Mid-line displacement if in water (how far the body is in or out of the water at different stages)
- Balance and gravity (e.g. leaning forward or to the side while running).

Exercises are easily understood if you divide the body into the broad sections—arms, legs, the trunk/waist and chest, and the head—and then classify each exercises into broad types of movements for each of these parts. For example, the legs might be used for walking or jumping. Within each of these two types of movement there is scope for a wide range of variations—for example, jumping could be done with the legs together or apart. Beyond this, different types of movements for one part of the body may be combined with different types of movements for

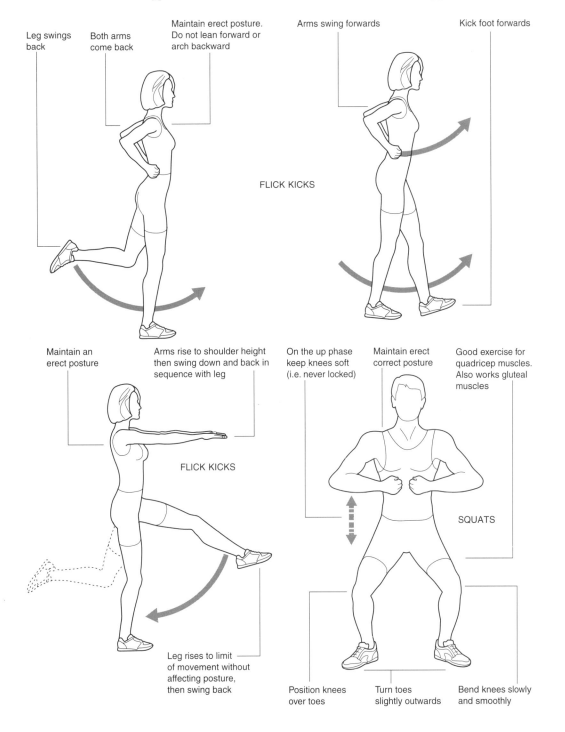

Leg swings back

Both arms come back

Maintain erect posture. Do not lean forward or arch backward

Arms swing forwards

Kick foot forwards

FLICK KICKS

Maintain an erect posture

Arms rise to shoulder height then swing down and back in sequence with leg

FLICK KICKS

Leg rises to limit of movement without affecting posture, then swing back

On the up phase keep knees soft (i.e. never locked)

Maintain erect correct posture

Good exercise for quadricep muscles. Also works gluteal muscles

SQUATS

Position knees over toes

Turn toes slightly outwards

Bend knees slowly and smoothly

another body part. The number of possible combinations therefore increases.

LEG MOVEMENTS

Moving the legs is more effective in getting the heart pumping than moving the arms, due to:

- Involvement of large muscle groups
- The distance from the heart—the muscles being worked are further from the heart, thus the extra blood needed for work must be pumped further
- Gravity—pushing blood back up to the heart goes against gravity, making the heart pump harder
- Legs weigh more than arms and therefore more effort is required to bring them into action and to sustain that action for extended periods.

For all these reasons, repeated energetic leg movements are the basis of most aerobic effective exercises—walking, running, jumping, stepping, cycling, skating, etc.

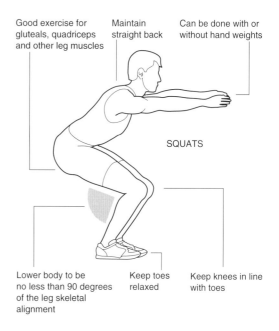

Good exercise for gluteals, quadriceps and other leg muscles

Maintain straight back

Can be done with or without hand weights

SQUATS

Lower body to be no less than 90 degrees of the leg skeletal alignment

Keep toes relaxed

Keep knees in line with toes

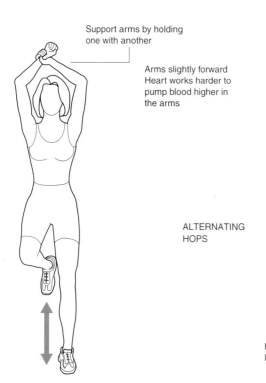

Support arms by holding one with another

Arms slightly forward Heart works harder to pump blood higher in the arms

ALTERNATING HOPS

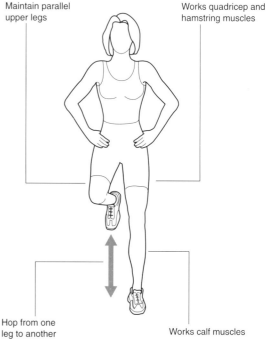

Maintain parallel upper legs

Works quadricep and hamstring muscles

Hop from one leg to another

Works calf muscles

Variations in leg movements are provided by:

- jumping jacks
- shuffles
- single leg lifts
- flick kicks
- dance steps
- squats
- lunges
- power walking
- jogging
- step ups
- hops/alternating hops

ARM MOVEMENTS

While most types of aerobic movements are based on leg movements, their effectiveness can be built on with the addition of arm movements to the exercise. Arm movements can vary in terms of intensity (to work the heart and muscles harder) and complexity (to increase interest, and/or challenge coordination skills).

Arm movements should complement the movements in the lower body, therefore avoid movements which make for difficult arm–leg coordination. For example, jumping jacks combined with alternating arm punches would be unnecessarily difficult to perform; lat raises or both arms moving together would work better. The sequence of arm movements should be a natural flow, and the speed and range of movement should be appropriate—in other words, avoid movements that are fast, stressful, high impact, confusing to follow/perform—arm movements should challenge but *not* confuse.

> Avoid arm movements above the shoulder for people with high blood pressure or shoulder impairment injuries.

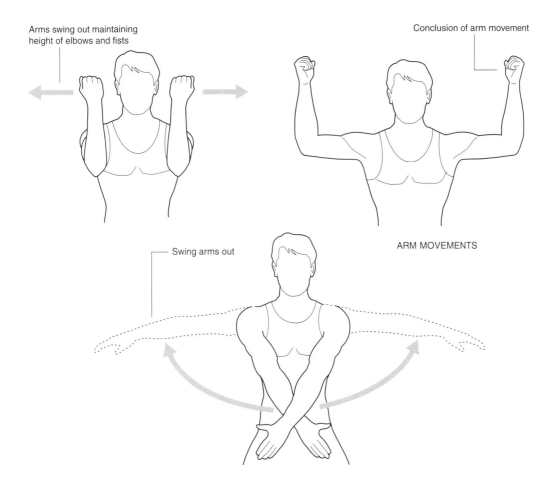

Arms swing out maintaining height of elbows and fists

Conclusion of arm movement

Swing arms out

ARM MOVEMENTS

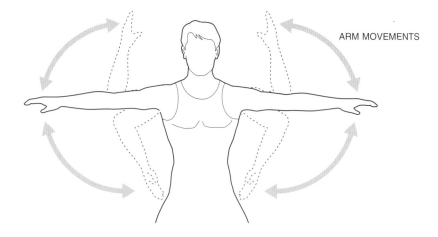

ARM MOVEMENTS

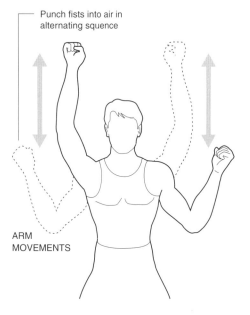

Punch fists into air in alternating squence

ARM MOVEMENTS

Avoid excessive repetition of the same movements. Variety of movement will provide balanced working of a wide range of muscles.

Arm movement variations might include:

- front raise
- side raise
- upright row
- low row
- reverse fly
- chest fly
- cross arms over chest
- bicep curl
- side curl
- side curl
- tricep extension
- chest press
- shoulder press
- lateral pull-down
- pump
- pump
- swing
- scoop

Arm movements can be used for a number of different leg positions. For example, sky punches (see left) can be combined with jogs, jumps, kicks, squats, single alternating leg lifts, steps, easywalk, etc.

RUNNING, JOGGING AND WALKING

Running and jogging differ from walking in three ways; they are faster, the gait is longer (the legs stretch further apart), and the work-out is more intense (more energy is burnt and the heart beats faster). Jogging is moving with a running gait (legs stretched) at a pace of between 60 and 90 seconds per 200 metres.

Many adults regularly walk for both fun and their health. Walking is low impact, with less stress on the joints and less injury risk than jogging or running. Even though walking is less strenuous than jogging, in a situation where all other conditions are the same (e.g slope, duration of exercise), walking can be a more valuable aerobic activity than jogging. The problem with jogging and running is that they place greater strain on the legs and jar internal organs and intervertebral discs more than walking does. Over a long period of regular jogging, a person is much more likely to suffer permanent injury than from walking.

Walking, jogging and running may look

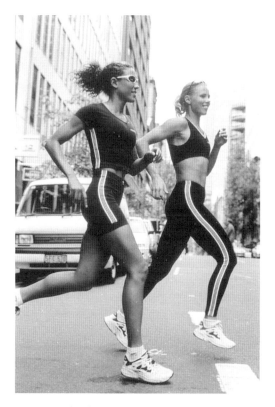

Jogging on hard pavement provides an excellent work-out, but if done consistently over many years often leads to joint damage, particularly in the knees. Wear suitable clothing and shoes.
PHOTO: COURTESY RUNNING BARE ACTIVE WEAR

like the simplest of activities, but as for any exercise there are good ways and bad ways of doing them. Common actions which may lead to injury or discomfort include:

- Poor rhythm
- Too much bounce
- Arms or trunk moving out of balance
- Trunk twisting or leaning too far forward
- Swinging the arms too much or too little
- Arms crossing over body mid-line
- Landing flat rather than rolling the foot
- Moving the foot or lower leg out to the side rather than straight forward
- Landing on toes.

Also, as a person ages some actions tend to change in walking:

- Feet are lifted less
- Pace becomes slower
- Strides become shorter
- Flexibility of the ankles is reduced
- Feet move with greater out-toeing
- Poor posture
- Over-use of hip flexors in the forward pelvic tilt position causes lower back pain.

WHERE TO RUN OR WALK

There are lots of options—in a gym on a treadmill, in a circuit inside a stadium, around an athletics or jogging track, on a fun and fitness trail, along a footpath, road edge, wilderness track, through a park, along the beach. Each of these has particular characteristics which might or might not make them a preferred option for you.

Points to consider include the surface, the number and steepness of hills, the distance and the rate of movement required to cover that distance in a convenient time period, the amount of protection from sun, wind, extremes of temperature, humidity, rain, and so on. Safety and security can be of particular concern for those running at night. The runner must wear clothing that makes them easily visible, the surface they run on should be smooth and visible to lessen the risk of tripping, and the route should be free of places where muggers might hide.

Surface The surface on which you run or walk must be considered. A hard surface such as asphalt or concrete causes greater jarring or impact upon the joints, hence an increased chance of injury. Some resilience or 'give' is advantageous—for this reason, choose artificial track surfaces or turf if possible.

Running or walking on sand in bare feet requires more effort and works the heart and leg muscles more than walking on asphalt, but can lead to foot problems. Sand does not provide the same support as a more solid surface, placing greater strain on foot muscles than similar exercise on a firmer surface. A slippery surface can also cause problems—you need grip both in your footwear *and* in the surface you are travelling over.

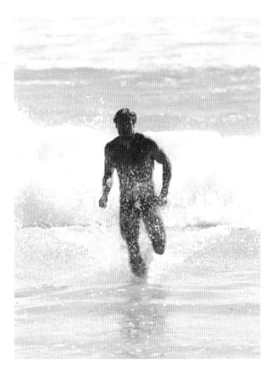

*Guy Andrews, Uncle Toby's Iron Man Champion.
Running on a loose surface (sand), or in shallow
water, requires more effort than on a firm surface.
For a very fit person, this can be an excellent
aerobic work-out, but for a beginner it is
inappropriate.*
PHOTO: COURTESY NO FEAR

Topography Running or walking up or
down slopes uses different muscles to those
used when moving over a flat surface. Uphill
work usually requires more effort from quadriceps and gluteal muscles. Going downhill uses
more eccentric contractions (i.e. contracting
muscles while lengthening), resulting in more
muscle soreness and a higher impact. Beach and
road running is often on a surface that slopes to
the side, which can place a lot of repetitive
strain on the knees, ankles, hips and lower back,
due to unbalanced side pressure.

Distance and movement rate The distance
you travel needs to be planned thoughtfully if
you are training outside. Determine the distance
you plan to walk and aim to maintain an even
pace over that distance, although for variety

you may wish to modify the pace from time to
time. If your course is very long, and you are
new at this type of exercise, keep the pace even
throughout and ensure you have access to
water. On your first few walks or jogs, be easy
on yourself or your class members—do not plan
for a marathon. Select an easy pace and a short
comfortable distance.

AEROBIC WALKING

A slow stroll for a short distance will not give
you a significant aerobic work-out, but a brisk
walk paying attention to body position will.
Make sure you are wearing comfortable shoes
with good support, and comfortable clothes.

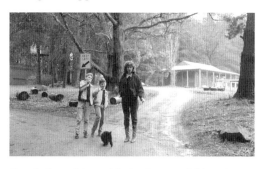

*Regularly walking with the dogs or children is one
of the most convenient and effective ways for
young adults to maintain their aerobic fitness.
They might not realise how important such
activities are to their general health and well-being.*

The body should always be upright, face
looking forward (not down), the heel should be
planted first and rolled before pushing off with
the toe, toes should face forward, not even
slightly sideways, shoulders should be slightly
back, arms should move in opposition to legs
(i.e. left arm moving backwards as left leg
moves forwards). This position achieves greater
stability.

Speed or power walking

You need a steady rhythm and a pace brisk
enough to raise a light sweat. The arms must
move as well as the legs. Take longer than
normal walking strides; in order to increase the
speed and energy expended you need to push

back hard on each step. Keep elbows bent and fists lightly closed. This can look silly, but put your ego aside.

A 10-minute power walk can be an excellent start to an aerobics work-out, while a 20- or 30-minute power walk by itself can be a great work-out.

This type of walking can require a little more motor skill coordination than other types, particularly if it is to be sustained for a full work-out period of half an hour or more.

Pole walking

This involves walking with two walking sticks (poles). It is the safest and perhaps best way to increase aerobic effort in a walk. The poles are used in a similar manner to ski poles. By pushing on the poles as you walk, the intensity of exercise is increased, and at the same time you are provided with greater stability. The poles work better if they have rubber bases to absorb any jarring.

A beginner walking this way at a rate of 4–5 km per hour gets a useful work-out. For more advanced training increase the walking rate to 6–7 km per hour.

Weighted walking

This involves carrying weights as you walk, either in your hands or attached to your body, usually as a weight belt. Excessive use of weights can, however, strain the parts of the body which support them, so be careful.

JOGGING

With most unfit people, jogging continuously will change an aerobic work-out into an anaerobic work-out (refer to Chapter 1). As the exercise becomes anaerobic, the person will not be able to continue, and hence will stop jogging.

A better alternative is intermittent jogging and walking—this can be done with or without a treadmill. Generally, beginners should jog for 100–200 metres, then walk for 50 metres, repeating this over and over for half an hour; or start with one-minute jog followed by a one-minute walk. Slightly fitter people might alternate a

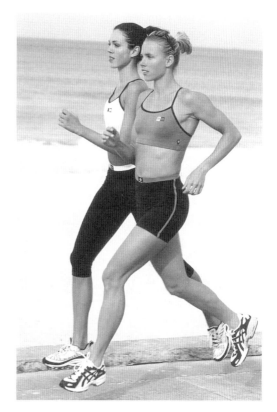

Jogging with a training partner can reduce boredom.
PHOTO: COURTESY RUNNING BARE ACTIVE WEAR

five-minute jog and two-minute walk. Adjust times and distances as fitness improves.

Advanced training can involve a faster rate of jogging over similar distances; lengthening the jogging segments, or an overall increase in the duration of the session, from a beginner's 25-minute work-out to perhaps 45 minutes to one hour.

Whatever you do though, stay within your limits. It is advisable to wear a heart-rate monitor and ensure that you do not exceed the recommended 75 per cent of maximum heart rate (MHR) for your age (MHR is calculated at 200 minus your age in years). MHR is now used to evaluate the effectiveness of interval training (say, one fast lap of an oval followed by one slow lap).

You can jog in all sorts of places—along streets, cross-country, on park tracks, around an oval, or on a treadmill. Fun and fitness trails are jogging tracks with exercise stations along their length to add interest and variety to the work-out. The concept is jog for a short distance, then undertake an exercise such as push-ups or chin ups, at the exercise station. By interspersing different exercises between bouts of jogging, the fun and fitness trail can create the same effect as alternating periods of jogging and walking.

CYCLING

Cycling is a popular and effective form of exercise but remember that you need to travel greater distances on a bike than you would doing a jog-walk-jog work-out. Cycling requires that you travel more than two to three times a jogging distance to achieve the same work-out. The intensity of the work-out can be controlled

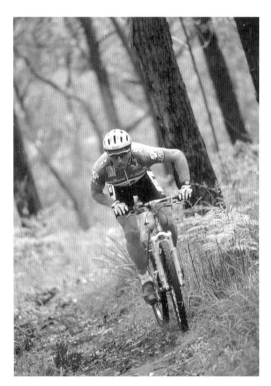

Rob Eva, Multiple National Mountain Bike Champion, maintains a high level of aerobic fitness through his bike riding.
PHOTO: COURTESY NO FEAR

by varying the workload, resistance, slope/grade, duration, distance, etc.

There are different ways of cycling, each with particular characteristics. For information on the different types of bikes see pages 25–26.

Cycling has several advantages:

- It is low impact, placing minimal impact on joints and ligaments
- It is good for beginners, the gears on mobile bikes and controls on stationary bikes allowing control over workload
- Mobile bikes can be used in interesting areas
- Stationary bikes are relatively quiet, especially compared to some treadmills, so you can watch TV while exercising.

To get the greatest benefit from riding a bike:

- The seat should be at the correct height—a too-low seat can put extra stress on knees and reduce performance, while a too-high seat prevents you achieving good pressure across bottom of pedal stroke
- Don't lock knees or ankle joints
- A too-high seat on a mobile bike can cause reduced balance control
- Toe-clips or toe-straps help to work agonist/antagonist muscles
- Always wear a bike helmet outdoors (it is law in some States)
- Good shoes are important for comfort and performance
- Use sun protection (appropriate clothing and sunscreen) when cycling outside.

Exercise bikes

Exercise bikes are stationary machines (they don't take you anywhere) which can be used inside. They have a number of advantages:

- You can ride under cover without getting cold or wet
- You can stop whenever you need to, and you don't need to get back home
- You can control the workload to achieve the duration and intensity of work-out you require

- You can vary the workload as and when you wish during a work-out.

Off-road bikes

Off-road riding generally provides a more strenuous work-out than other cycling exercises. A one-hour mountain bike ride can provide a better work-out than a three-hour road ride. Off-road riding's main attraction, however, is that it puts fun and variety into a work-out.

SWIMMING

Swimming can be either competitive or non-competitive. Swimmers of all ages have always trained to improve fitness and compete, but today an increasing number of people are swimming regularly for no reason other than to maintain their own fitness.

The health advantages which swimming offers include:

- Very low-impact exercise in still water (higher impact in surf)
- Very meditative (psychologically relaxing)
- Useful for maintaining aerobic fitness when other muscles are strained.

Consider also:

- Swimming can be anaerobic if you sprint, so don't go too fast
- Different swimming styles work different muscles, so mix the styles during a distance swim to reduce fatigue
- Rhythm is important—swim steadily and use both arms and legs equally; some kick-board work helps balance a work-out
- Waterproof heart monitors can be useful.

Note: The cooling effect of water results in a heart-rate around 10 beats per minute less than from an equivalent work-out on land.

Swimming programs

Swimming programs can be designed to motivate participants in ways as diverse as the imagination allows. This might include setting goals and rewards appropriate to and achievable by the participants involved.

Fitswim, a scheme developed for non-competitive swimmers in Australia, emphasises group training, aiming to remove the boredom often experienced in lap swimming (hence increasing motivation). It provides challenging but achievable incentives and goals.

A Distance Challenge might involve attempting to progressively swim a particular distance (maybe 5 km, 10 km, or even the width of the English Channel). Each participant swims laps over any number of visits, recording their cumulative distance until their goal is reached. Upon reaching their goal, a prize might be awarded (e.g. a certificate, free entry to the pool for a specified period).

Most public swimming pools have amateur and masters swim clubs, and both private and group coaching.

ROWING

Rowing can be done on a rowing machine (stationary), or in a canoe, boat, surf ski or board. Rowing has the advantage over some other forms of aerobic activity that it spreads the effort across a wide range of muscles, giving a fuller aerobic work-out, especially if the seat is on sliding rails to allow more use of the legs. It provides a good break from running and is very low impact.

It is essential to row properly, keeping in mind the following pointers:

- Start slowly until you perfect your technique
- Keep the back straight, work the legs (it is easy to just work the arms, thus putting too much strain on the back and resulting in back injury)
- Do not bring the knees up too close to the chest as you stroke—this can force the arms to work harder as you lose the ability to push hard with the legs.

Rowing offers many benefits:

- It is an excellent aerobic work-out
- It exercises all main muscle groups
- It is time-efficient
- It relieves stress

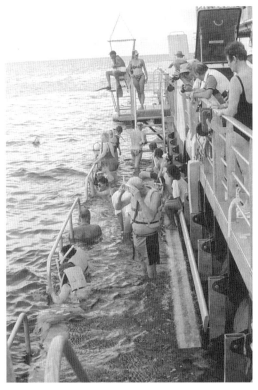

Virtually any type of water activity is a good low-impact aerobic work-out—even snorkelling on the Great Barrier Reef.

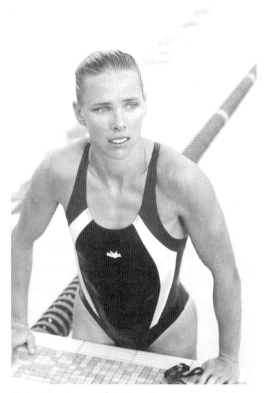

Swimming is one of the best low-impact aerobic exercises you can do.
PHOTO: COURTESY RIVAL SWIM/TRIATHLON WEAR

- Rowing machines are built to be low impact, and foster rhythmic movement
- Many rowing machines have meters to provide feedback so that monitoring the work-out is possible.

Rowing in a boat involves working against air (air resistance contributes to a low-impact work-out). There are three parts to the rowing action:

1. The catch, when you move the arms forward—this works the shoulder, triceps, back, abdominals, hamstring and calf muscles.
2. The drive, when you start to pull back—this works biceps, forearms thighs, calves, hamstrings, back and buttocks.
3. The finish—this works the abdominals, thighs, calves, buttocks, forearms, biceps, shoulders and sides.

As a general rule, for an 'average' person 2 km of rowing equals around 1 km of jogging, in terms of the aerobic work-out achieved. These figures can vary greatly, however, depending upon a person's weight and the level of fitness in the upper body and the lower body.

STEPPING AND CLIMBING

Climbing might be achieved through using a stepping machine in the gym, a raised platform in step class, by walking up a hill or mountain, walking up steps, as in a tall building, or by rock climbing. On a machine or in a step class you climb up and down in alternate steps, but in other situations you may climb up a great distance before you come down. These differences result in use of different muscles in different ways. Rock climbing or walking a mountain can place greater stress on muscles, and without due care is more likely to result in fatigue or injury.

Step machines

Both step machines and rock climbing require a fair degree of skill. Non-mechanised stepping machines in particular require a good deal of coordination.

Mechanised (computer-controlled) machines help establish and maintain rhythm and an appropriate level of effort.

The steps of a stepping machine *must* be parallel to the floor. Railing must be stable, and ergonomically designed. If you use a stepping machine for an extended period, it is important to introduce variety into the session. If the foot pedals are wide enough, you can move your feet periodically into different positions. You might begin the work-out with the feet flat on the pedals and pointing straight in front. You might then move the feet to the edges of the pedals; you can shift your weight more onto the balls of the feet, or more onto the toes. For a heavier work-out, you may hold weights, if your coordination is very good, you can even stand on a stepper backwards.

Always stretch before using a stepping machine, and always warm-up and cool-down with more gentle movements at the beginning and end of a session.

SKIPPING

Skipping a rope can form the basis of an effective aerobic work-out. It does require a degree of concentration and physical coordination to avoid getting tangled in the rope; but once some basic skills are mastered, many variations can be developed to add interest and challenge to a work-out.

Skipping has a number of advantages:

- It doesn't require expensive equipment (e.g. like a treadmill or cycle ergometer) . . . you only need a skipping rope!
- It works the arms as well as the legs

- It requires greater coordination and concentration than jogging or cycling and can be useful for developing these qualities.

Minimising impact

Skipping can be a particularly high-impact exercise, so it is not advised for people with injuries, arthritis or other problems. A cushioned surface is preferred, particularly for an introductory class.

Skipping can be high intensity and high impact from the moment the skip commences, so a warm-up doing something other than skipping is advisable.

If skipping for any extended period, intersperse periods of skipping with periods of stretching, particularly stretching the lower back, hip flexors, calves, tibialis anterior, shoulders and hips.

Impact is minimised by using the proper landing technique—landing on the balls or toes of the feet and then allowing the heel to touch the ground; bracing the abdominal muscles also reduces impact on the lower back. Landing on the toes alone will cause calf muscle fatigue and knee problems.

Equipment

- Use a lightweight rope
- Wrap tennis racquet tape around handles to improve the grip if necessary
- Towelling wrist bands will prevent sweat dripping onto the handles and making them slippery
- You may wish to wear long leggings and a full T-shirt to avoid the risk of accidental whip-mark injury
- Wear shoes with good support (ball and fore-foot cushioning are particularly important)
- Double-tie shoelaces.

Skipping classes

Participants in skipping classes skip rhythmically to a set beat (126 beats per minute (bpm) is appropriate). Beginners should do an introductory class to learn the basics before attempting a standard class.

Participants should be far enough apart to allow for the movement of the rope, with extra space allowed for exercisers who have difficulty staying in the one position. Form up the class in staggered lines, so that no-one stands directly behind or in front of anyone else.

Keep knees and ankles flexed, never fully locked, to better absorb impact.

Stress that participants should never let go of a rope—flying ropes and handles can readily cause injury.

Cross-country skipping

Once your coordination is good enough you can try skipping along a jogging track or trail. Be aware of other people and obstacles, though. You need an even surface, and clear space above and to the sides of where you move.

Variations
- Try holding a conversation while you skip—this challenges your concentration and can help develop better coordination
- Develop controlled breathing patterns while skipping
- Try landing on the same foot twice or three times before going to the other foot; but not more than four times, as the repeated impact can be dangerous.

Beware: Moving your head in different ways while skipping can be dangerous to your neck and/or shoulder muscles and joints.

Jump Rope for Heart Scheme

This is a scheme operated in Australia by the National Heart Foundation in association with the Australian Council of Health and Physical Education (ACHPER). It promotes skipping primarily through schools, maintaining a registration scheme, and providing various resources such as teacher's manuals, skipping ropes, posters, T-shirts, stickers (for students), and fundraising materials.

See the directory in Appendix VIII for ACHPER's contact details.

BALL SPORTS

Some ball sports are better for aerobic fitness than others. Playing an appropriate sport regularly can be part of your regular aerobic fitness program, but always remember that you need to exercise three times a week. Playing any sport once or twice a week, even for an extended period, is still not adequate.

Soccer

This is a particularly vigorous sport which, depending on the intensity of play, can provide a very good aerobic work-out. It is, however, high impact, and can easily over-strain leg muscles, particularly if you are involved in other intense training programs at the same time.

Tennis, squash and racquet ball

All these ball sports use similar muscle groups, but the work-out intensity varies. Tennis, which focuses on short sprints interspersed with very little activity, can be good for building certain muscles, but is a relatively poor aerobic work-out. If you are relatively fit, a game of squash or racquet ball can provide a much more appropriate aerobic work-out. Because all these games involve lots of stopping and starting, they are all relatively high impact and risk injury. If they are played at an intensity appropriate to your level of fitness and capability, they can be very effective aerobically.

Aussie Rules, rugby and gridiron

Football sports such as Aussie Rules and rugby are similar to soccer in terms of exercise benefits, but not as good as soccer. Gridiron is particularly poor in terms of aerobic benefits. The potential of impact is higher in these sports, with the risk of damage more serious.

Basketball and netball

These two popular sports have periods of high aerobic activity interspersed with periods of low aerobic activity. Over the duration of the whole game players get a very good work-out in cardiovascular terms. Short jarring movements are the biggest disadvantage.

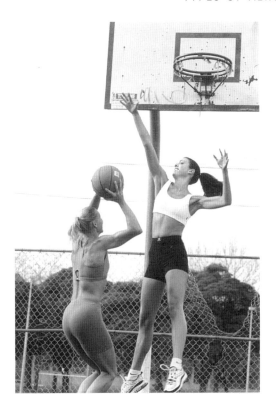

Basketball is an excellent aerobic work-out.
PHOTO: COURTESY RUNNING BARE ACTIVE WEAR

Hockey
Hockey rates close to soccer in terms of aerobic activity.

Water polo
Water polo provides both great aerobic and anaerobic work-outs. It also has the benefit of being a great leg work-out. All water sports are generally low or no impact.

Cricket, golf, croquet, lawn bowls
These sports are generally considered low in aerobic benefits when compared to other more active sports.

Rock climbing
Due to endurance and strength required to maintain climb, this exercise necessitates high aerobic fitness.

SURFING
Depending on the ability of the surfer, usually the back and arm muscles are worked hard when paddling out; the legs and postural muscles are worked when surfing in. The aerobic effect is much greater if the waves are bigger, and the activity is continuous, otherwise surfing can tend to be more anaerobic.

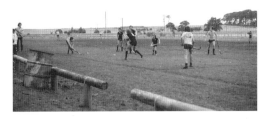

Hockey is an excellent sport for maintaining aerobic fitness.

Volleyball
Possibly close to basketball and netball in terms of health benefits. The surface on which the game is played (indoor hard-court or outdoor sand-court) will dramatically affect aerobic activity, muscle activity and the risk of joint problems.

HORSE RIDING
Certain types of equestrian sports are better for aerobic fitness than others. Cross-country, dressage, jumping, polo and polocrosse can be good aerobic work-outs, but a high level of riding skill is required for horse riding to be an aerobic exercise. Trail riding and learning to ride are a more balanced form of exercise.

The more active equestrian sports require a greater amount of work and training on the part of the rider, using gluteals, legs, back and abdominals, as well as postural muscles. It can be very aerobic.

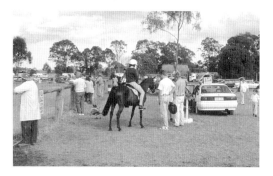

Some types of horse riding can provide a good aerobic work-out; horse riding, however, requires a high level of skill if it is to be tackled as an aerobic activity.

SKATING

The benefits of skating, in all its forms—ice skating, in-line blades, rollerskates, skateboarding—are similar to those of jogging or power walking, with the added bonus that the postural stabiliser muscles are worked for balance.

In-line skates, skates and skateboards have inbuilt resilience or shock absorption; they can provide low-impact exercise, but because of the speeds involved there is also greater risk of bodily harm if you take a fall.

The surface needs to be smooth and predictable for safety. Think also about the safety of people around you. Do not skate dangerously close to them or use them as cushioning when you fall. Additionally, as both the walking public and skaters tend to use the same areas, you need to be considerate of their mobility.

For the sake of your body, wear safety gear. This can include:

- Helmet
- Knee and elbow pads
- Wrist protectors or gloves
- Sunglasses to protect from sun glare and UV light
- Sunscreen lotion if outdoors for extended periods of time.

What are the benefits of skating? Skating on in-line rollerblades at a speed of 9–10 kilometres per minute is equivalent to running at 19–20 kilometres per minute.

Variation

Ways in which you can vary skating as an aerobic exercise include:

- In-line skating (i.e. holding onto several people in a line); this can be gentle, social and an effective aerobic work-out
- Cross-country skating
- Figure skating
- Skating in a rink, or bowl, etc.
- Skating on a skateboard, rollerblades, or conventional rollerskates.

SKIING

Cross-country skiing is both an endurance activity and a great aerobic work-out. While it uses many of the same muscles as running, it can actually increase oxygen intake more than running does. Indoor ski machines can provide a reasonable substitute work-out.

The benefits include working the hamstrings, calves and lower back muscles; using poles works the arms and shoulders, particularly when climbing up slopes. For a work-out benefit similar to running, you need to ski for approximately twice as long.

With all sports that incorporate speed there is an element of risk. The unpredictability of terrain on the ski-fields significantly contributes to the frequency of injury.

Grass skiing can provide a similar level of benefit without the costs of travel and accommodation on the ski fields. Grass skiing is done on grass or artificial-surface ski slopes, using skis with tracks which looks a little like the tracks on a bulldozer or army tank.

JUMPING

High jumping and long jumping on their own are not aerobic activities; but jumping combined with running can provide an excellent aerobic work-out. This can involve hurdling on the

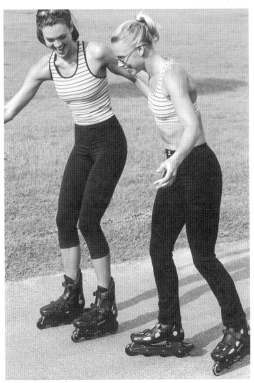

In-line skating (rollerblading) has become very popular for recreation. It promotes good aerobic exercise and leg muscle development.
PHOTO: COURTESY RUNNING BARE ACTIVE WEAR

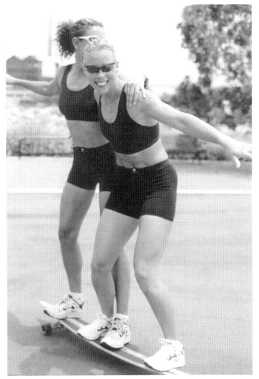

Skateboarding is a popular and excellent aerobic exercise, but without protective gear and appropriate technique, accidents are relatively common.
PHOTO: COURTESY RUNNING BARE ACTIVE WEAR

athletics track, or cross-country running in which you jump fences and other obstacles.

Jumping can be used as a component of other exercise regimes. The act of jumping does have the potential to cause a lot of harm to joints if technique is poor and the landing surface is hard. For jumping to be used properly, it is important to land on a resilient surface, land in a way that minimises any impact on the body, and combine the jumps with lower-impact movements so that any stress is not repetitive.

Jumping can be very beneficial as a warm-up for running, hurdles, long and high jumps, boxing, marathon running and other sports.

Where jumping is incorporated into a training program, it is essential that the participants be carefully instructed in the correct action, and that the moves are both carefully considered and appropriate to the fitness level and needs of the participants.

TAI CHI (TAI QI)

This slow form of Chinese meditative exercise is a surprise to most aerobic participants. The secret is combining movement with deep diaphragmatic breathing to allow the heart to reach a target heart-rate without strenuous activity. The beneficial effect of Tai Chi on health can be put down to the way it increases the efficiency of the heart's pumping action by enhancing the relaxation mode of the heartbeat, whereas Western medicine tends to emphasise the contracting mode of the heartbeat. The leg movements incorporated in the various Tai Chi postures aid the pumping mechanism of the circulatory system, a benefit mentioned previously in other aerobic exercises.

There is no jarring or other harmful side effect in Tai Chi. The emphasis on body posture and balance ensures minimal strain. Although the rhythmical movements are easy to learn, proper instruction is necessary to ensure they are done correctly for maximum benefit. Various styles of Tai Chi work the limbs and heart at different workloads within a time-frame ranging from five minutes to 25 minutes. It is recommended that movements be repeated in the prescribed sequence for 20 minutes or longer at least three times a week. Devotees perform Tai Chi every day, safe in the knowledge that no harm can be done if movements are performed in the right way.

EXERCISING IN WILDERNESS AREAS

Some types of aerobic activities can take you into isolated terrain or wilderness areas, raising special considerations. Above all, you need to be sure that it is permissible for you to legally and safely enter the areas you plan to visit. You may require a permit to enter or to undertake a certain type of activity.

Safety in the wild

Never go into isolated areas unaccompanied—always take a partner with you; stick to established routes, particularly if you are a beginner; carry a small First Aid kit; a mobile phone and drinking water; wear appropriate clothing, i.e. protective gear and footwear; and carry materials for basic repairs for bike riding, canoeing, or other equipment-based sports activities.

EXERCISE CLASSES

Exercise classes include gym work-outs, aerobics, dance, step, pump, outdoor and aquarobics, among others. Participants may do one type alone, or combine various classes over a period of days or weeks. There are no set combinations which must be followed, however. The following types of classes are most common. Some of these class types can overlap benefits for the participants.

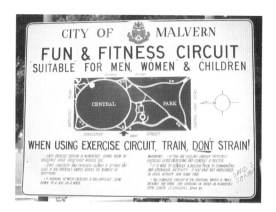

Fun and fitness trails through parks can provide an excellent facility for regular exercise, but signage explaining how to make the most of them is very important.

Any form of exercise will assist in improving your fitness for a specific activity. There is a definite amount of cross-over benefit in aerobic activities, but you still get the most benefit from your efforts in the particular activity that you are training for. For example, an endurance swimmer might be very fit for swimming, but would not be as aerobically fit for cross-country skiing.

LOW INTENSITY

(also called Gentle, Beginners, Introductory and Light)

These classes are intended for all types of people, but most commonly for beginners, those with below-average levels of fitness or those in need of rehabilitation.

Intensity: Low to medium.

Facilities needed: None necessary, apart from music equipment. Light weights or low steps are optional.

Music rate: 124–148 bpm in aerobic phase.

Movements: Controlled, safe and balanced moves, no complicated choreography.

Comments: Confidence-building, usually fat-burning, easy and safe.

EXTENDED

(also called Advanced)
Intended for healthy people with above-average fitness.

Intensity: High.

Facilities needed: A surface with good grip, excellent ventilation, low temperature (to minimise overheating), music equipment.

Music rate: 145–165 bpm.

Movements: Intense, can be highly choreographed combinations.

Comments: Necessary to incorporate continual challenge and motivation.

LOW IMPACT

Low-impact aerobics require at least one foot to be in contact with the ground at all times.

Intended for beginners, older people, injury rehabilitation, pregnant women.

Intensity: Low/medium.

Facilities needed: A surface with good grip, excellent ventilation, low temperature (to minimise overheating), music equipment.

Music rate: Approximately 145 bpm.

Movements: Choreographed, well taught and interesting.

Comments: Instructor needs to be a good motivator as low impact can become boring and participants usually need encouragement to work hard.

STEP

(also called Step Reebok)
Step classes can be designed to suit almost any level of fitness or coordination.

Intensity: Low, medium or high.

Facilities needed: A surface with good grip, excellent ventilation, cool temperature (to minimise overheating), music equipment.

Music rate: 118 bpm for beginners to 128 bpm for advanced.

Movements: Can be basic to highly choreographed combinations of moves.

Comments: Safety needs to be considered with turns, lateral movements, etc.

The founders and leaders of the step concept were the Reebok organisation, hence step classes are commonly referred to as 'Step Reebok'. There is a great deal of variation possible in step classes, including the intensity and degree of motor skill coordination required, duration of the class, height of step, etc.

- *Step Reebok* (also called Introductory Step, Step Basics) is aimed at beginners, intermediate and advanced.
- *Step Athletic* can suit a wide range of people, but is more strenuous, without being particularly complex—you don't need particularly high levels of coordination, but usually do a higher number of repetitions.
- A *Step Moves* class has more challenging and complex sequences of moves, requiring greater concentration and physical coordination in combination with physical exertion. This type of class can be medium or higher intensity according to the type of participants and their needs.

Music speed and step height
- For the novice who hasn't exercised much recently—approx. 120 bpm onto a 10 cm step.
- For someone who exercises regularly, but hasn't taken a step class before, music at 124 bpm and a 15 cm step.
- For the average regular step class participant—20 cm step; music at 126 bpm.
- For the skilled, regular step class participant—25 cm step, music at 128 bpm.

How to step
Movements should not see the foot/knee loaded when pivoting—that is, when a turn is performed, the leg should be airborne to allow unstressed rotation of the knee and foot.

Participants should not step off the front of the block. This puts too much load on the knee joints.

As with all aerobic exercise, the abdomen and lower back should remain firm, with the body in an upright position while stepping.

The step action should see the entire foot

placed on the top of the step, with gentle (low-impact) movements.

The knees, hips, shoulders and head should all be over the feet when on the step.

Don't step at a height which forces the weight-bearing knee to flex more than 90 degrees; about 60 degrees is preferable. At 90 degrees, the step is too high.

NEW BODY

(sometimes called Muscle Conditioning or Shape Up)

This type of class is aimed at working muscles to increase muscle tone and flexibility through low-impact moves, with hand weights. The heart-rate is raised throughout to keep the body warm as the muscles are stretched and toned; but should not be raised excessively. The low-impact simple moves are designed for upper body conditioning.

This class is suitable for all.

Intensity: Low to medium.

Facilities needed: Hand weights, 2 kg or less.

Music rate: 70–136 bpm.

Movements: Low impact, usually using hand weights.

Comments: Usually used as a body tone, muscle endurance class. Low impact due to using hand weights. Safety considerations important.

DANCE

(can include Jazz and Body Beat)

Incorporates dance moves such as funk, Latin, jazz or street dance.

Suitable for anyone, but easier to do if participants have some natural rhythm, i.e. a good understanding of music and beat.

Intensity: Variable.

Facilities needed: Flat floor surface, preferably a suspended floor.

Music rate: 127 bpm or higher.

Movements: Movements can be complex, requiring a relatively high level of motor skill coordination.

Comments: Can be fun and challenging.

HI-LO

(also called Combo)

Combines high- and low-impact exercises into the one class.

Suited to intermediate-level exercisers.

Intensity: Medium to high.

Facilities needed: No equipment required. Hi-Lo is faster than 'New Body', which utilises hand weights.

Music rate: 145–165 bpm.

Movements: Usually choreographed for variety and to maintain interest.

Comments: Gives people the option to work at high/low impact when they are ready. Similar to interval training, where a period of high heart-rate activity is alternated with a period of low-impact recovery.

INTERVAL

Combines periods of more strenuous activity with periods of less strenuous activity.

The body is slowly warmed up through an introductory phase; after which the heart-rate is raised to a high but safe level; the heart-rate is then lowered and sustained at a level higher than the resting rate, but not a particularly high rate, leading to a recovery phase, then the heart-rate is raised again . . . etc.

Interval classes suit participants with medium to high levels of fitness.

Intensity: Medium to high.

Facilities needed: A surface with good grip, excellent ventilation, cool temperature (to minimise overheating), music equipment, hand-held weights are optional (the amount of weight depending on the level of fitness).

Music rate: 145–160 bpm.

Movements: Varied.

Comments: Can be choreographed or repetitive moves depending on the type of class and participants.

PUMP

Pump is a licensed program, available in Australia only through Les Mills. It involves a planned sequence of moves using a barbell.

Pump can suit any level of fitness or motor skill; only a minimal level of coordination is required.

Intensity: Can be adapted to the individual by increasing or decreasing the amount of weight placed on the barbell.

Facilities needed: Barbell and weights.

Music rate: 115–125 bpm.

Movements: Stationary.

Comments: A good introduction to a class situation. No coordination skills required.

CROSS TRAINING

(also called Combo, Hybrid or Medley)
This type of class involves combining different styles of exercise class.

Usually suited to the fit individual.

Intensity: Adaptable.

Facilities needed: Depends on the type of cross training (e.g. steps, hand weights, etc.).

Music rate: 124–145 bpm.

Movements: Variable.

Comments: Used for variety.

CIRCUIT EQUIPMENT CLASS

(also called Body Titan, Body Torque)
A popular type of class used to increase aerobic fitness. The different names all refer to basically the same thing. A circuit class is held in a room set up with exercise equipment which is intermixed with running, skipping and aerobic-based exercises to increase fitness and body strength. The machines usually utilised in this class are Keisers, which are isotonic-based, providing resistance throughout the entire range of movement, both concentric and eccentric.

These classes are excellent for beginners wanting to increase their knowledge about exercising before entering the gymnasium with a resistance program. They also allow participants to get used to the exercises and build general strength. Many of the machines and exercises are similar to machines used and exercises performed in the gymnasium

setting—for example, rowing machines, steppers, treadmills, bicep curls, tricep extensions, squat machines, upright row and bench presses.

OUTDOOR CIRCUITS

These include Fun and Fitness Trails, medicine ball circuits, water circuits, dumbbell or bar circuits; continuous circuits. They are intended for participants with a medium to high level of fitness.

Intensity: Varies with the equipment, usually self-motivated.

Facilities needed: Usually park circuits supplied by clubs or local government authorities.

Music rate: Either the participants' own headsets (Walkmans), set at an individual pace; or none.

Movements: Vary on each piece of equipment.

Comments: Good for variety; it can be healthy to exercise out of doors in a park where oxygen levels are usually higher and more conducive to aerobic activity. Dependent on weather and self-motivation. Safety can sometimes be of concern: location, design and construction are all factors which need to be considered before using an outdoor circuit. Requires maintenance by the responsible authority, which is not always done.

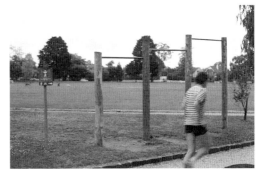

Fun and fitness trail station: Chin-up bars beside a running track provide an optional exercise station for joggers.

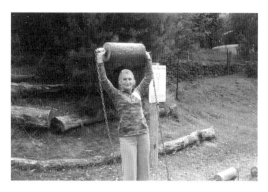

Fun and fitness trail: A weight-lifting station with weights attached to the ground by chains.

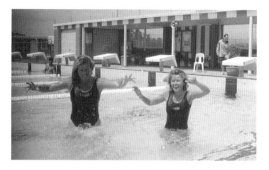

Water aerobics is best carried out in water about waist-deep.

DEEP-WATER RUNNING

Due to the reduced impact level, deep-water running is excellent for older people, injured people in rehabilitation, or anyone doing a lot of exercise, such as professional sportspeople, who are at risk of impact injuries from other forms of exercise.

Intensity: Low to high.

Facilities needed: A pool or other safe body of water at least 2 metres deep; float belts for buoyancy.

Music rate: 124–136 bpm, or none (some groups, often older people, may prefer no music).

Movements: Usually leg and arm movements, primarily variations on running and cross-country skiing actions.

Comments: A very safe way to increase aerobic fitness.

For more information on deep-water running, consult *Aqua Fitness*, also by John Mason (Kangaroo Press, Sydney, 1999).

WATER AEROBICS

Due to the reduced impact level, water aerobics classes are excellent for older people, injured people in rehabilitation, or anyone doing a lot of exercise, such as professional sportspeople, who are at risk of impact injuries from other forms of exercise.

Intensity: Low to high.

Facilities needed: A pool or other safe body of water 1.2 to 1.5 metres deep.

Music rate: 124–156 bpm.

Movements: Varied—all areas of the body.

Comments: A safe and effective work-out for most people.

SWIM PROGRAMS

An excellent form of interval training for competent swimmers.

Intensity: Can be adapted to the individual by increasing or decreasing the rate and distance.

Facilities needed: Goggles are advisable in chemically treated water to protect the eyes.

Music rate: None.

Movements: Varied, but mainly upper body.

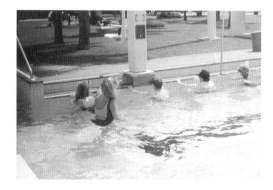

After an aerobic work-out in water, stretches can be carried out holding onto the edge of the pool for stability.

Comments: Safe form of cardiovascular training with low skeletal impact. Some people who have swum laps excessively over many years report neck problems caused by constantly holding the head up to see where they are going. The likelihood of such problems occurring will be minimised if the swimming technique is good. This is where an expert swimming coach can be an advantage.

STRETCHING

Any type of exercise session should begin and end with stretching as part of the warm-up and cool-down periods. Stretching as a warm-up allows the muscles to prepare for exertion by increasing blood flow within the muscle. Likewise, at the conclusion of exercise, stretching allows the body to circulate blood and oxygen back to those areas that are now lacking. Stretching, done slowly, controlled and completed properly, will significantly reduce the likelihood of injuries occurring during exercise, reduce the likelihood of soreness after exercise, and help increase flexibility.

Aerobic warm-ups are recommended before commencing stretches and full-on aerobic exercises. The temperature of the muscles should be raised before engaging in stretching exercises through a number of gentle warm-up exercises such as walking or jogging. Stretches that can be performed after a warm-up are discussed below.

BODY STRETCH

Phase: This should be the first of your warm-up stretches or the last of your cool-down stretches.

Starting position: Stand with the feet shoulder-width apart and with knees slightly bent.

Description: Reach skyward with both arms. Grasp the left wrist with the right hand and give a gentle pull toward the right. You should feel a stretch along the left side of your arm, shoulder and abdomen. Hold for 5–10 seconds, then repeat with the right arm. Perform this stretch at least twice.

Variation 1: Side stretch—gently sweep the arms in a sideways arc down to the sides of the body, then rest the hands on hips and perform a mini-lunge, bending the left leg and keeping the right stationary, while swaying the hips to the left. A gentle stretch should be felt in the left hip and the inner thigh of the right leg. Alternate the move, shifting left to right, repeating the lunge 3 to 4 times for each leg, and hold for 10 seconds. Finish the overall stretch by loosely shaking the arms and legs. See figures on page 60.

Variation 2: One-arm stretch. See figure on page 60.

Precaution: Maintain good posture.

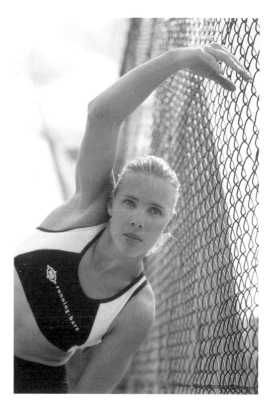

Stretching is essential before and after exercise routines. Appropriate clothing should not restrict stretching movements.
PHOTO: COURTESY RUNNING BARE ACTIVE WEAR

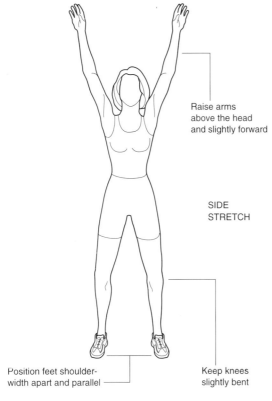

Raise arms above the head and slightly forward

SIDE STRETCH

Position feet shoulder-width apart and parallel

Keep knees slightly bent

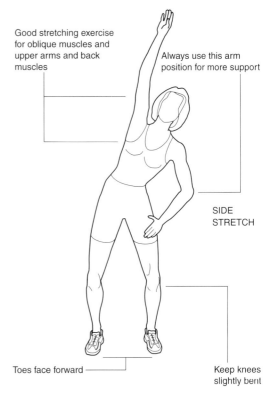

Good stretching exercise for oblique muscles and upper arms and back muscles

Always use this arm position for more support

SIDE STRETCH

Toes face forward

Keep knees slightly bent

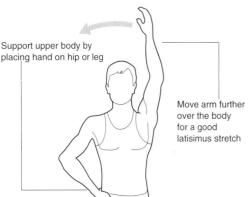

Support upper body by placing hand on hip or leg

Move arm further over the body for a good latisimus stretch

ONE ARM STRETCH

Place feet shoulder-width apart, toes facing forward

Bend knees

GLUTEAL STRETCH

Phase: Warm-up and/or cool-down.

Starting position: Lying down, feet flat on the ground with both knees bent.

Description: Keeping the left knee still bent, use your left hand (or both hands) placed under the right knee to pull the right knee towards your body. Keep right knee bent. Once a gentle pull is felt, hold for 10 seconds. Repeat with the left leg and perform the entire exercise up to three times per leg. This stretch is also very gentle for the back and is ideal for those who suffer from back pain.

Note: When the raised leg is bent (flexed), the gluteals are stretched. If the raised leg straightens, the hamstrings will get a stretch.

Variation 1: Try the same type of movement in the standing position. Aim to bring the knee up to the chest towards the opposite shoulder and hold for a count of up to 10 seconds.

Variation 2: Reclining gluteal stretch—this movement is done to the side and provides good support for the body. See figure on page 61.

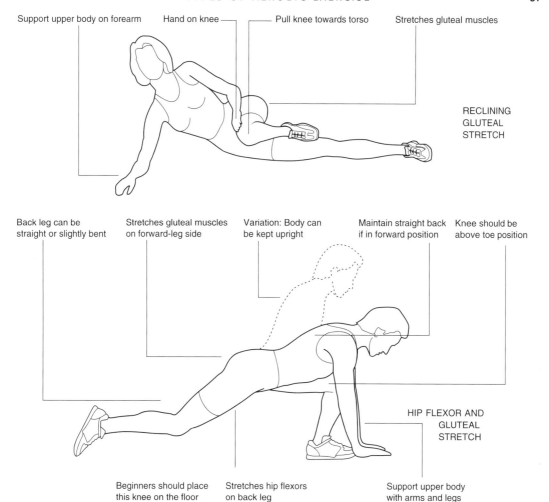

Support upper body on forearm | Hand on knee | Pull knee towards torso | Stretches gluteal muscles

RECLINING
GLUTEAL
STRETCH

Back leg can be straight or slightly bent | Stretches gluteal muscles on forward-leg side | Variation: Body can be kept upright | Maintain straight back if in forward position | Knee should be above toe position

HIP FLEXOR AND
GLUTEAL
STRETCH

Beginners should place this knee on the floor | Stretches hip flexors on back leg | Support upper body with arms and legs

Variation 3: Combined movements, like hip flexor and gluteal stretch (see figure above in a lunge-like position, provide one exercise that stretches more than one muscle group at a time.

Precaution: Maintain a straight back. Do not allow the lower back to curve while lying down.

LUNGES

Phase: Warm-up and/or cool-down.

Starting position: Stand up straight with your feet placed shoulder-width apart and hands resting on hip.

Description: Step to the side with the left foot, bending the left knee while keeping the right foot stationary and shifting the hips to the left. You should end up with the left side of the body aligned and the right leg off at an angle. You should also feel a gentle pull on the inner thigh of the right leg. Keeping the feet in place, shift the hips and body to the right, bending the right knee and straightening the left.

Repeat this process, shifting from left to right, repeating up to 3 times each side, and hold for 10 seconds.

Variation: Increase the intensity of the movement by adding arm movements. As the body is shifted left, allow the arms to drop down by the sides, then swing in an arc across the body, stopping when the arms are level with shoulders. When swinging the arms to the right (while body is shifting left), the right arm should finish fully extended, at shoulder height and pointing to the right of the body. The left arm should be bent at the elbow, with the forearm pointing right and stretched across the chest. Repeat this process, swinging in the opposite direction to the lunge.

Precaution: Be aware not to strain the inside of the thigh. Take the stretch to where it feels comfortable.

HAMSTRING STRETCH

Phase: Warm-up and/or cool-down.

Starting position: Stand up straight with both feet together. Hands on side of thighs.

Description: Keeping the left leg straight and foot in place, step backwards with the right foot and bend the right knee while simultaneously bending from the waist (not the lower back). Lower the body until you feel a gentle pull at the back of the leg. Hold for 10 seconds, then repeat the process with the right leg. Repeat 3 times for both sides. See figure on right.

Variation 1: Flexing the toes of the forward foot upwards, which involves stretching the calf muscle and gastrocnemius, provides a variation

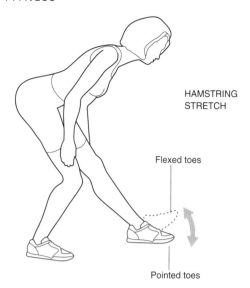

HAMSTRING
STRETCH

Flexed toes

Pointed toes

to the move, although it may interfere with the hamstring stretch.

Variation 2: Do the lying-down gluteal stretch described above but with a straight leg raise.

Variation 3: Seated hamstring stretch—this movement is good for beginners. See figures on this page and page 63 (more advanced version).

Precaution: Maintain a straight back, try not

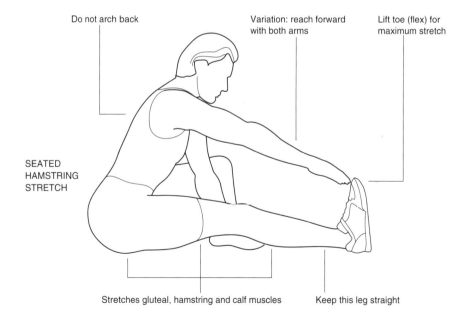

Do not arch back

Variation: reach forward with both arms

Lift toe (flex) for maximum stretch

SEATED
HAMSTRING
STRETCH

Stretches gluteal, hamstring and calf muscles

Keep this leg straight

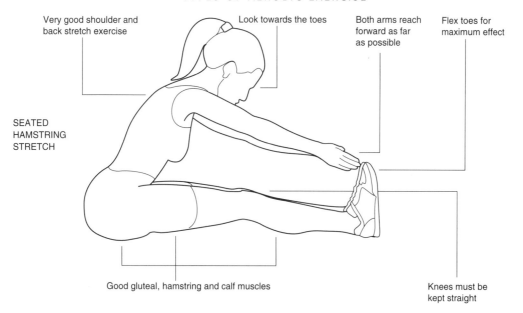

Very good shoulder and back stretch exercise

Look towards the toes

Both arms reach forward as far as possible

Flex toes for maximum effect

SEATED HAMSTRING STRETCH

Good gluteal, hamstring and calf muscles

Knees must be kept straight

to arch the back. Do not overstretch the hamstring when doing variation 2.

QUADRICEP STRETCH

Phase: Warm-up and/or cool-down.

Starting position: One foot on ground, other leg held in hand behind buttocks, knees close together.

Description: Hold for 10 seconds, stretching thigh muscle.

Precaution: Knees together, buttocks tucked under, back straight.

GROIN/ADDUCTORS STRETCH

Phase: Warm-up and/or cool-down.

Starting position: Stand with legs apart and knees turned outwards.

Description: With hands on knees, push the knees further out to one direction, feeling the stretch on the inside of the legs.

Precaution: Keep the back flat and feet in line with the knees.

ADDUCTOR STRETCH

Phase: Warm-up and/or cool-down.

Starting position: Stand near a wall or support with one hand against the support. Cross left leg over in front of the right leg.

Description: Place the sole of the left foot against the floor, then try to pull the foot against the floor back in the left direction. Gently push left hip outwards. A stretch should be felt in the upper outer left leg.

Precaution: Do not push hip out too much—a gentle stretch should be felt.

PECTORAL, DELTOID AND BACK STRETCH

Phase: Warm-up and/or cool-down.

Starting position: Standing straight with feet shoulder-width apart and knees relaxed, raise arms horizontal, straight out to the sides, making the body into a 'T'.

Description: With feet firmly planted, sweep arms forward, keeping them straight and fully extended, gently rounding the shoulders, until they meet at the front of the body. Grasp the wrist of one arm and give a gentle forward pull,

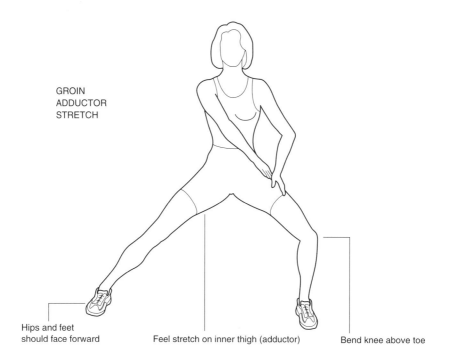

GROIN ADDUCTOR STRETCH

Hips and feet should face forward

Feel stretch on inner thigh (adductor)

Bend knee above toe

feeling the stretch right across the arms and shoulders. Repeat this with the other arm. Then release the grasp and swing the arms back, until they are reaching as far behind the body as possible. The arms may lower in height and some people may be able to touch the hands together behind the back. You should feel a stretch right across the chest. Then bring your arms back to the starting 'T' position. Repeat at least 3 times. Make sure you retain good posture while swinging the arms backwards.

Variation: Additional to this, class participants can pair up and assist each other—one person stands behind the other providing a resistance with their hands against the other's arms while they push forward.

Precaution: Maintain a good posture while swinging the arms backwards. Some people may stretch too far behind their back to join their hands and cause an unnatural pull, especially if the head is poked forward.

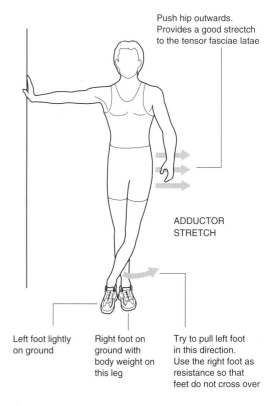

Push hip outwards. Provides a good strectch to the tensor fasciae latae

ADDUCTOR STRETCH

Left foot lightly on ground

Right foot on ground with body weight on this leg

Try to pull left foot in this direction. Use the right foot as resistance so that feet do not cross over

SHOULDER/DELTOID STRETCH

Phase: Warm-up and/or cool-down.

Starting position: Legs apart and knees slightly bent. Stretch left arm across the body towards the right at shoulder level. Grasp left arm just above the elbow with the right hand and pull toward the body until a stretch can be felt in the left shoulder and shoulder-blade. Keep the head turned towards the left shoulder. Hold for 5–10 seconds, then repeat the process with the right arm. Repeat the whole exercise a minimum of 3 times.

Precaution: The arm being pulled across the body must be kept straight. Posture is important. This stretch should be pain-free; if it hurts, do not continue.

TRICEPS STRETCHES

Phase: Warm-up and/or cool-down.

Starting position: Stand straight with feet flat and knees flexed.

Description: Lift the left arm straight above your head, then bend at the elbow, touching left shoulder. Reach over the head with the right hand and grasp the left elbow, then push gently down until you feel a gentle stretch through the upper arm and shoulder-blade. Hold for 5–10 seconds, then repeat the process with the right arm. Repeat the whole exercise a minimum of 3 times.

Precaution: Keep the hips pushed forward and bottom tucked under so the back does not arch.

CALF STRETCH

Phase: Warm-up and/or cool-down.

Starting position: Facing a wall or other solid structure, press both hands against the wall, about shoulder height.

Description: Keeping hands in place, bend the left knee and step back with the right leg, keeping that leg straight, but without locking the knee. You should be in a lunging position. Lean body toward the wall until you feel a gentle pull in your calf. Hold this stretch for 10 seconds, then step forward and repeat the process, but with opposite legs (right knee bent, left leg back). Repeat 3 to 5 times for each leg.

Variation 1: Bend your back knee a little, creating a stretch behind the ankle.

Variation 2: In the push-up position and one knee on the ground, push the heel of the other foot backwards while its toes are still connected to the ground. See the figure below.

Precaution: Ensure posture is maintained.

LOWER BACK (ERECTOR SPINAE) STRETCH

Phase: Warm-up and/or cool-down.

Starting position: Stand with legs shoulder-width apart.

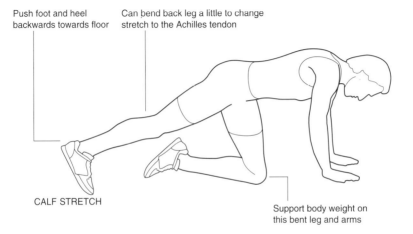

Push foot and heel backwards towards floor

Can bend back leg a little to change stretch to the Achilles tendon

CALF STRETCH

Support body weight on this bent leg and arms

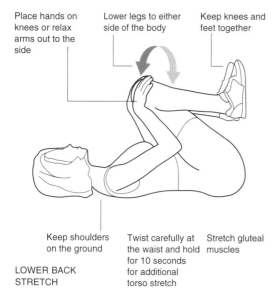

Place hands on knees or relax arms out to the side

Lower legs to either side of the body

Keep knees and feet together

Keep shoulders on the ground

Twist carefully at the waist and hold for 10 seconds for additional torso stretch

Stretch gluteal muscles

LOWER BACK STRETCH

Description: Rotate the body (go to one side and hold, then go to the other side, with care), looking behind the body and trying to touch the backside with the hands.

Variation: Lie on the floor and bring knees up to chest supported by the hands. Gently rock from one side to the other in order to lower the legs to either side of the body. Twist at the waist.

Precaution: Only rotate as far as the body allows, being careful not to strain the neck or back; do not use as repetitive twisting.

MUSCLE CONDITIONING

Muscle-conditioning exercises are often carried out at the same time as stretching to strengthen certain muscles which can be associated with postural and other problems if they are too weak. Problems are more likely to develop during aerobic exercise if these muscles are not strong enough.

Three of the most useful types of exercise

in this group are push-ups, back arches and abdominal exercises.

PUSH-UPS

There are three different ways in which push-ups can be done, used according to the level of fitness and muscle strength.

Level 1 is the easiest, and most appropriate for a beginner or an older person with poor fitness. It is performed on the knees and hands with the bottom in the air. The chest is moved towards the floor, keeping the abdominal muscles tight. The back should be kept straight—avoid any significant arching at all times. This ensures that the muscles of the chest region are being used correctly.

Level 2: The body is straighter, but the participant is still on the knees. The entire upper body from the hips to the shoulders goes towards the floor in a straight, tight, position.

Level 3: Only the toes and hands touch the floor, and the body should be kept in a straight line, held tight. This should only be attempted by individuals strong enough to support their own weight through the chest and abdominal muscles.

BACK ARCHES

Lie on the floor face down with the left hand under the forehead. The right arm lifts up with the left leg, keeping the hips on the ground. This is performed slowly, and in a controlled fashion, and repeated on the other side.

For the beginner the repetitions would be only 5 or 6, where a fitter person might do 10 or 20.

An alternative back-arch exercise starts with both hands under the chin; keeping the legs and hips on the floor, attempt to lift the head and chest off the floor slowly, hold for a couple of seconds, then lower. This movement is repeated a number of times.

Keep feet together Pivot at this point Maintain a straight back Use the arms to lower just the shoulders and chest

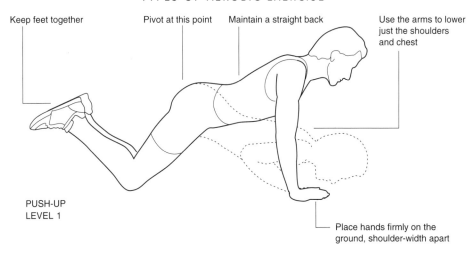

PUSH-UP LEVEL 1

Place hands firmly on the ground, shoulder-width apart

Keep feet together Pivot at this point Keep back straight The entire upper body is lowered to the floor

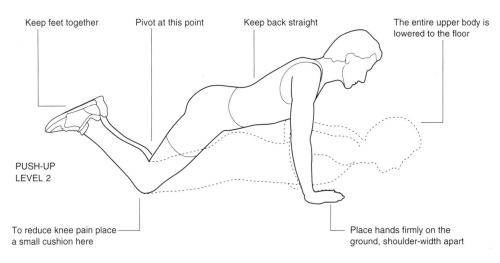

PUSH-UP LEVEL 2

To reduce knee pain place a small cushion here

Place hands firmly on the ground, shoulder-width apart

Maintain straight back Entire body is lowered to the ground

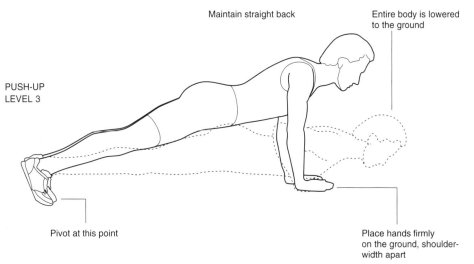

PUSH-UP LEVEL 3

Pivot at this point

Place hands firmly on the ground, shoulder-width apart

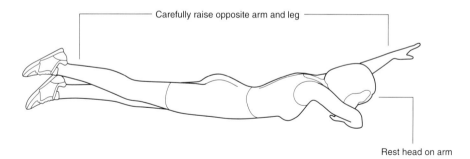

Carefully raise opposite arm and leg

Rest head on arm

BACK ARCHES

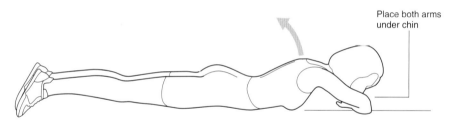

Place both arms under chin

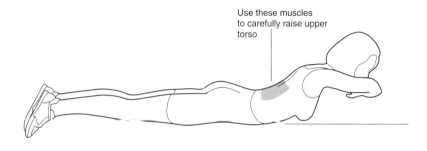

Use these muscles to carefully raise upper torso

ABDOMINALS STRETCH

Lie on the back, with the legs bent (knees off the floor), and the feet flat on the floor. The hands are clasped together and placed behind the lower part of the head and neck to support the neck. The eyes are towards the roof, and the head is held in a neutral position. There should be *no* pull on the neck, nor any rapid movements which might damage the neck.

The body is lifted up until the shoulderblades are just off the floor. If the upper body is lifted higher than halfway, the hip flexor muscles, rather than the abdominals, are beginning to be worked. Hip flexors that become too tight can create back problems.

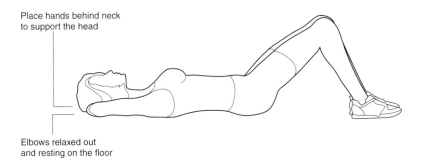

Place hands behind neck
to support the head

Elbows relaxed out
and resting on the floor

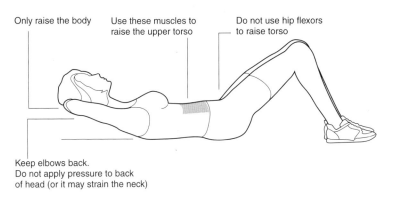

Only raise the body

Use these muscles to
raise the upper torso

Do not use hip flexors
to raise torso

Keep elbows back.
Do not apply pressure to back
of head (or it may strain the neck)

ABDOMINALS

CHAPTER 4

SPECIAL PEOPLE AND SITUATIONS

Aerobic exercise should be tailored to meet the needs of the individual. Persons who are not fit and exercise only sparingly should undertake relatively low-intensity, low-impact and short-duration exercise. In contrast, a person with above-average fitness needs to exercise for longer periods at a higher intensity to maintain or improve aerobic capacity.

There are many people, however, who require special consideration due to unique factors which can impact on undertaking aerobic exercise—people who have a temporary or permanent condition, either physical or physiological, which affects what types of exercise they can or should do.

Medical clearance is advised for all groups of people who may be considered at risk—for example, older people, those who are pregnant, have prior medical problems, disabilities, are overweight, etc.

PREGNANCY

Women may still wish to participate in aerobic exercise during both pre- and post-natal periods.

In the early stages, and throughout most pregnancies, aerobics can still be performed, with the proviso that it is advisable to reduce intensity and in some cases avoid specific exercise routines. It is easier to conduct an entire lesson with women at the same or various levels of pregnancy than to try to teach a lesson with women who are both pregnant and not pregnant. Low-impact aerobic activities are most suitable.

The aerobic instructor working with pregnant women needs to keep the following in mind constantly:

- Heart-rate should be regularly monitored and kept within safe limits.
- Body temperature should be monitored—participants must not get too hot.
- Flexibility may be limited as pregnancy advances; conversely, due to hormonal activity there is greater than usual elasticity in ligaments and tendons, so care needs to be taken here.
- Comfort is paramount.
- Pelvic floor problems may develop, so take care with the types of exercises which affect pelvic floor muscles.
- Excessive aerobic activity can create reduced oxygen levels in the body, possibly reducing oxygen supply to the baby.

Avoid the following activities:

- Exercises in the third trimester that require good balance
- Dehydration at all times, but in particular during the first trimester
- Supine positions
- Activities that may cause strain or trauma to the abdominal region—this covers a number of sports
- Extreme environmental activities such as mountain climbing and scuba diving
- High-impact sports and activities
- Movements that cause jarring to the body.

Pregnant women who suffer from any of the following conditions are recommended not to exercise:

- History of pre-term labour
- Incompetent cervix

- Pregnancy-induced hypertension
- Pre-term rupture of membranes
- Persistent bleeding during second and third trimesters
- Breathlessness.

Need for referral to specialists when limits are reached

It is important that pregnant women see a medical doctor before and throughout the period if they take part in aerobics. A specialist doctor may advise individuals not to perform specific movements or suggest that they take an easier low-impact class.

Benefits

The significant benefits of exercise for pregnant women include shorter periods of labour, less incidence of complications during pregnancy, labour and delivery, and generally fewer symptoms of nausea, fatigue, leg cramps, poor body condition, poor sleep and backache.

Good education is the first step in ensuring the safety of the individual. Secondly, the frequency, intensity, time and type of aerobic exercise is extremely important—pregnant women have to understand how to modify their exercise program. The pregnant exerciser needs to know not only what she is doing but why. There can be serious implications for women who do not alter their routine and it is essential that the growing baby be the most important consideration.

Participation in aerobic or aqua aerobic exercise in the early stages of pregnancy should occur at a frequency that the person is comfortable with and used to. As the pregnancy progresses the frequency and intensity should be trimmed down to eliminate any possible discomfort or early childbirth. It is also important to realise that during pregnancy hormones are released that loosen ligaments, so care should be taken not to overstretch when exercising to prevent injury.

It is vital that the intensity of the session does not force the heart-rate to exceed 145–155 beats per minute, as rates higher than this can result in adverse effects on the baby. Higher heart-rates in some pregnant women have been shown to cause foetal stress. The resting heart-rate rises naturally during pregnancy, therefore the amount of exercise required to increase the heart-rate will be less than in the non-pregnant woman. It is suggested that a pregnant woman should wear a heart-rate monitor during exercise to establish how long it takes to reach the recommended maximum heart-rate and to allow her to stay at 145–155 bpm or lower, depending on fitness and age. Continuous safe exercise for 25 minutes with a heart-rate of 145 bpm should have no adverse effects on the baby in a normal healthy pregnancy.

The type of exercise that the pregnant exerciser engages in is important. Sporting activities which are not recommended include gymnastics, basketball, horse riding and surfing, which carry the risk of harming the baby through a hard blow to the abdomen, repetitive twisting or turning, or a fall. Low-impact aerobic exercises are a safe and relaxing activity if completed in the correct manner.

To modify a routine for pregnant women:

- Use non-stressful exercises involving major muscle groups
- Allow enough time for exercise or form changes
- Avoid trauma against the floor or any other equipment that may be used
- Decrease the amount of repetitive twisting or turning movements performed.

Aerobic exercise machines that are generally safe for the average healthy pregnant woman include rowing machines, stair climbers and treadmills.

Some of the better specific exercises to perform include shoulder shrugs and rotations, pelvic floor exercises, pelvic tilts and rocks and abdominal curls (only in early pregnancy). The aim should be to condition muscles that support and strengthen posture.

OLDER ADULTS

There are several obvious limitations for older persons in a class or exercising individually. An older person generally has more fragile bones

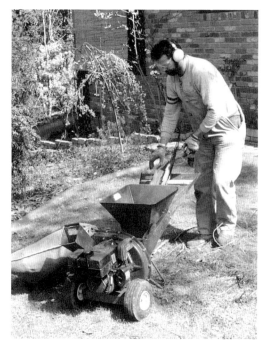

If you aren't a 'gym person', you can keep aerobically fit in other ways. Working in the garden, or doing odd jobs around your home, can provide just as good an aerobic work-out as going for a jog, or riding an exercise bike.

and skin, and reduced aerobic capacity, compared to a younger person. Their exercise needs to be modified accordingly. Older people should be advised to have medical clearance before entering an aerobic exercise program, and to renew that medical clearance every six months. Older adults are more likely to suffer from such conditions as diabetes, heart disease, deterioration in hearing, eyesight or coordination, and osteoporosis and arthritis. Instructors should take these conditions into consideration when planning an exercise program.

Older adults often participate in exercise for physical and socialisation reasons. The exercise session should be kept non-stressful and utilise major muscle groups. Exercises should be designed to mobilise, strengthen and improve flexibility. Instructions should be given clearly and slowly, allowing enough time for exercise or form to change.

Osteoporosis

Osteoporosis, the development of increasingly fragile bones, is a condition mainly of older people. Poor eating habits, smoking and other lifestyle factors can make the condition worse in some older people than others. The deterioration process can be slowed through exercise and using the body. Water exercise, such are aqua-fitness classes, is safer for anyone with osteoporosis. Aerobic fitness programs can also help—movements such as jumping and jarring should be avoided, however, and all movements should be performed at a slower pace than in a young adults class. Sufferers from osteoporosis benefit from the action of gravity during exercise such as walking.

Arthritis

Rheumatoid arthritis Occurs when the synovial membrane in a joint becomes thickened and inflamed. This can occur in people of any age.

Osteoarthritis Caused by the normal wearing of joints throughout a person's lifetime. As such it tends to occur in older people.

Vigorous exercise can aggravate arthritic conditions, but mild and gentle exercise can be beneficial, increasing lubrication of the joints during warm-up. If the exercise program is pleasant for the participant, then the intensity of the program is good; if the exercise program is painful, it is best to reduce the intensity. There are different types of arthritis; but the exercise recommended for each type is generally the same.

Arthritic people should take twice the normal time for the warm-up phase of a program. Take longer to do stretches, but avoid any stretches which are particularly painful.

If performing aerobic programs in water, arthritic people must avoid cool water, exercise only in warm water, ideally around 30–31°C, doing gentle exercises.

CHILDREN

Relatively few limitations apply to children exercising in a class, or individually. Children usually have better flexibility, and are in better general condition, than most adults; however, they are smaller, so equipment and other facilities will need to be scaled down accordingly. Children are also often less conscious of the risks involved in different physical movements, largely due to their lack of life experience, hence safety may be an issue requiring extra attention.

There is only a need for referral to specialists where a child is diagnosed with, or suspected to have, a particular medical condition.

Children are very active by nature and have a shorter attention span than adults. Consequently, a teacher in aerobics needs to utilise the energy produced while maintaining attention and interest. Children are generally regarded as a safe risk category, but a few considerations must still be met in a safe and caring way.

Factors that may hinder participation include asthma and weaknesses in muscle tendons, joint structure and growth plates. Body temperature should be monitored throughout the exercise program just as for adults: children can also suffer from heat exhaustion, and more easily than an adult. Children are more likely to suffer hypothermia, especially in such things as water sports and snow skiing, due to having less body mass per surface area.

Aerobics can be used to aid children's physical development, gross motor skills and fitness. It is extremely important that activities be kept fun, energetic and safe. While providing a variety of activities to forestall boredom, the instructor needs to remember to keep instructions simple and concise, use encouragement and positive feedback, and create a fun and challenging environment.

Important points to remember about children's activities:

- Incorporate games to maintain attention and interest.
- Keep games fun and active.
- Keep children moving.
- Safety is extremely important—keep an eye on all children all the times, and be qualified in teaching this age group and in First Aid.

PEOPLE WITH DISABILITIES

People with disabilities are limited in class participation or exercising individually—this is very individual, depending on the type of handicap. Physically handicapped people have obvious restrictions to movement of certain parts of the body. A paraplegic, for example, must rely on movement of the arms to increase the heart-rate, given that the legs do not move. Swimming or wheelchair sprinting can achieve this. Remember that activities which are challenging for a handicapped person could be boring for an amputee or a paraplegic.

It is advisable for disabled people to have medical clearance, usually from a physiotherapist, before undertaking an exercise program. Activities generally need to be specifically tailored to each individual.

Wheelchair access needs to be considered when catering for the physically handicapped.

Mentally handicapped
A mentally handicapped person may have full movement of the muscles, but may find complex exercise routines impossible to co-ordinate and perform. Activities need to be repetitive, fun, motivating and easy to follow. Aqua aerobics are probably the best, safest and most successful type of aerobic activity for mentally handicapped people.

Epilepsy
It is advisable to have parents or helpers available to assist, as medical emergencies such as seizure, fainting and anxiety attacks can be relatively common. Excitement, music or even flashing or flickering lights can trigger a seizure.

OVERWEIGHT PEOPLE

Exercise opportunities for overweight people may be limited by the size of equipment. Excessively obese people may simply not fit into a machine, or be too heavy for an exercise machine.

People who are overweight but not excessively obese do not usually need medical clearance to exercise unless they are over 35 years of age. If they have a particular medical condition, though, it is advisable to seek medical advice before undertaking an exercise program.

Problems for obese people include:

- Embarrassment, especially if using equipment which is difficult to get on and off, or which exaggerates their weight (e.g. sitting on a small seat on an exercise bike).
- Jarring can occur because there is so much weight moving about; movements should be low impact.
- Overheating: cool loose-fitting clothing such as shorts and T-shirts is recommended.
- Diabetes: this is a medical condition which requires clearance from a doctor. Diabetics must eat before exercise.
- Heart disease: these are medical conditions which require clearance from a doctor. It is advisable to wear a heart monitor and avoid working at higher than the 60 per cent **training heart zone**.
- Ideally, in order to burn fat it is best to maintain an exercise program at 60 per cent of **maximum training heart zone**.

It can be dangerous for overweight people to undertake excessive exertion. In an aerobic exercise program it is important to modify the movements and intensity to suit the participants. If done carefully, aerobics can be suitable for anyone who is overweight, but they should not exercise hard. Obese people are best to exercise at a lower intensity for longer—sessions of at least 30-minutes. Start with three sessions per week, perhaps increasing to four once the exercise is becoming more comfortable.

Be careful not to cause overheating. Full and gradual, even extended, warm-up and cool-down periods, are very important. A slight increase in heart-rate will be a great benefit to the overweight person so there is no need to overdo the work-out. The instructor should remind overweight exercisers to drink plenty of water.

A lot of encouragement and motivation is needed.

OTHER HEALTH CONDITIONS

Allergies

An allergic reaction involves the body acting abnormally to some external factor, such as a chemical, food or airborne particles such as dust or pollen. Certain plants, such as privet and many grasses, are a relatively widespread problem when in flower. Cigarette smoke can also affect some people badly. These common problems should be kept as far as possible away from exercise classes.

In some rare instances, individuals can actually be allergic to exercise. Such a problem may manifest in a skin rash or occasionally swelling in the throat or face (exercise-related urticaria), which can persist for hours after exercise. Affected individuals can suffer low blood pressure, breathing difficulties, or even shock and unconsciousness, due to exercise-related allergy.

Asthma

Asthma involves narrowing of the air passages carrying air into the lungs, which by restricting air flow makes breathing difficult. This narrowing can be caused by a build-up of mucous and/or contraction of muscles surrounding the air passages. Although asthma is not fully understood, what is known is that the following things can cause an attack:

- Allergic reaction (e.g. food additives, pollen or dust in the air)
- Infection
- Physical stress
- Emotional stress.

To minimise chances of an attack, asthmatics must be conscious of their condition, always take time to warm up slowly and not persist with exercise if there is a heightened risk (or any sign) of an attack. Any chance of ill-effects can be minimised by lengthening the duration of the warm-up and cool-down periods. Given that some foods can trigger an asthma attack, it is best that asthmatics avoid eating for two hours prior to exercise. Aerobic exercises that excessively increase cardiorespiratory function can create problems for anyone with a respiratory problem. Milder forms of exercise like swimming, aqua aerobics or deep-water running are generally the best forms of exercise for severe asthmatics.

Approximately 10 per cent of the Australian population is considered susceptible to exercise-induced asthma, which can be defined as some form of breathing difficulty due to bronchial constriction and muscle spasms occurring during exercise. If you are asthmatic, or are instructing someone in this 10 per cent, you should take the following precautions:

- Take longer to warm-up than is normally recommended—a 5- to 10-minute warm-up should last for at least 15 minutes.
- Avoid exercising in poor-quality air—polluted city air, stale air in an air-conditioned building, air contaminated with pollen from blossom or grass.
- Increase fitness levels gradually.
- Avoid exercising when you or the person you are instructing is in poor health, e g. if either of you has a cold.
- Breathe through the nose rather than the mouth, particularly if the air temperature is cold.

Anaemia

Anaemia is simply a lack of haemoglobin in the blood, often accompanied by a reduced number of red blood cells. This results in tiredness, lack of energy, breathlessness and the skin can become pale in colour. The most common cause is a lack of iron; which in turn may be caused by an inadequate diet, or through blood loss (anaemia can be more common in women who lose more blood than the average during menstruation). Adolescents and vegetarians are a little more prone to anaemia than the general population. Iron supplements in the diet can correct the problem, but as extended use can result in iron toxicity, the degree of supplementation should be carefully watched.

It has been shown that people like professional athletes, who exercise frequently, can suffer lower than normal levels of ferritin (a substance that stores iron reserves in the body). This is called 'sports (induced) anaemia'.

Diabetes

Exercise can affect the physiology of a diabetic. Most experts suggest that a diabetic should eat some fruit or bread before exercise, and something else after exercise. A diabetic should check with a doctor before entering into any regular exercise program. It may also be necessary to drink something like diluted fruit juice during a session. If any signs of hypoglycaemia (decreased blood sugar levels) are noticed, exercise should be stopped.

Hypoglycaemia is indicated by:

- A dry tongue
- Hyperventilation
- Rapid and weak pulse
- Intense thirst and frequent urination
- Constipation, muscle cramps and altered vision.

Fibromyalgia

People with this illness have constant aching of muscles, and consequently do not sleep well. They are often very cautious about undertaking any exercise. There is no cure, but there are treatments to manage and minimise the pain. Regular exercise can improve blood flow to muscles and also help. As posture can deteriorate with this condition, maintaining good posture during exercise is important.

Gentle exercise is appropriate for sufferers of this condition. A gentle walk program can start with 5 minutes each session for three sessions or more a week, extended by maybe 1 or 2 minutes each week, until 20 minutes each session is reached. A warm-up and cool-down incorporating some gentle stretches is essential.

CHAPTER 5

SAFETY

Safety is an extremely important aspect of any exercise activity. Safety considerations include:

- The condition of the facilities or site being used (i.e. exercise areas, toilets/locker rooms, access, etc.)
- The types of exercises being carried out
- The equipment being used.

AEROBICS CLASSES

Aerobics classes are generally conducted with numerous participants. The more people in the room the more dangerous it can be. Tripping, banging into walls and coming off a step onto someone else can all make the class dangerous, or even just annoying, for the participants and the instructor.

It is essential that each participant have sufficient space in which to extend their limbs to the fullest extent, and to travel if required. A class with many people may be great motivation for the clients, and be more cost-effective to run, but it is harder work for the instructor, who must be constantly scanning for any problems.

SAFETY-RELATED ISSUES

INCORRECT EXERCISES

If clients are not constantly monitored and corrected, it is easy for incorrect movements to become common practice in an aerobic workout. Many exercises and stretches are well known as potentially dangerous, while current research is always providing us with updates as to which stretches and exercises are, and are not, suitable for different situations.

Important points to remember about exercises typically used in fitness regimes are:

- In any movement where the knee bends forward, ensure that the knee does not go over and past the toe. This places excess pressure on the knee and can cause injuries.
- Constant impact and stress on the lower limbs (e.g. more than a certain amount of running/aerobics per week) can cause many injuries. Stress fractures, also known as shin splints, tendonitis, Achilles tendon problems, and knee injuries caused by poor alignment of the knee with the lower leg, can all play a part in causing problems. Some of these can be corrected with rest, a visit to the podiatrist with orthotics being prescribed, or by physiotherapy. These complaints and injuries have to be carefully monitored by the individual and the fitness leader.
- Lower limb problems can also cause back pain and associated problems. Poor alignment in one part of the body can create problems in other areas distant from that part.

See Chapter 3 for information on correct technique for a range of different exercises and stretches.

SAFETY IN OTHER AEROBIC ACTIVITIES

The wide variety of activities that may be considered as aerobic activity make it very difficult to provide detailed lists of safety precautions for each one. There are some general rules that should be considered for all activities:

- Use the correct equipment, and ensure it is in good condition. This could range from properly fitting shoes, with soles suitable for the conditions they are being used in, to wearing bright, reflective clothing that is easily seen (especially for runners using the roads) to protective helmets (whitewater canoeists, cyclists).

- Avoid unnecessarily dangerous situations such as busy roads, poor weather, poor visibility (at night, foggy conditions), dangerous water conditions (for sports such as swimming, canoeing, surfing).

- Don't overdo any activity. Try for gradual increases in the intensity and duration of any aerobic activity being undertaken.

- Instructors should be aware of any health conditions that participants may have; participants must be honest about any health problems, and obtain the relevant medical clearance.

- Participants should be aware of their own personal limitations and exercise at a pace that is comfortable and appropriate to their needs. A suitable level of exercise can be determined in consultation with an experienced instructor, and where appropriate for those with existing health problems, a medical practitioner.

FIRST AID

Teachers of aerobic activities should be certified in First Aid and Resuscitation, and registered as an Aerobics Instructor with the relevant association (i.e. AFAC).

Whether exercising in a gym, at home, or elsewhere, it is always wise to have someone else nearby who can help in the case of emergency. Even a very fit person can have an accident, fall, sprain an ankle, or develop a cramp.

The Australian Fitness Accreditation Council (AFAC) monitors the standards of fitness courses and practitioners in Australia. Other countries may have similar bodies, with similar training requirements. The existing minimum training (at the time of printing of this book) for aerobic teachers in Australia to be registered with AFAC is the Aerobics Instructor Course which covers Fitness Leaders Core Theory, plus Aerobics module and First Aid certification.

For other aerobic type activities it is necessary to obtain advice from the governing body, if one is available, for the level of expertise required to conduct classes in each activity or sport. In general, it is recommended that for any outdoor activity at least one person present has a recognised first-aid qualification from a body such as the Red Cross, St John's Ambulance, the Australian Sports Medicine Foundation or the Royal Life Saving Society.

In addition, for fixed facilities such as gyms, staff need to be well informed about the facilities where they are working, and acceptable procedures. They should be taken through an initial training/orientation period when they first commence work; and review sessions should be conducted at regular intervals, particularly when any changes are introduced.

Ideally, the First Aid room should be clearly identified, well lit and ventilated, with a non-slip washable floor, good access to toilets, and be large enough to rotate a stretcher 360 degrees. It should contain washing facilities, lockable cupboards, two chairs, an examination couch/bed, a stretcher, telephone, a waste container/rubbish bin, resuscitation masks and rubber gloves.

The location of First Aid facilities should be clearly signposted, but access to such a facility should be controlled (e.g. accessed only through the reception area), with only authorised staff having free access. Patrons requiring First Aid treatment should be accompanied by an authorised staff member at all times. Larger facilities, those catering to 300 or more people at any one time, should have supervisory staff trained in First Aid to an advanced level. In some cases they may be required to employ a registered nurse. First Aid kits should be kept complete, and checked regularly, with items replaced as soon as they are used or become out of date. Provision could also be made to have an Emergency Vehicles Only parking area in a suitable location, perhaps outside the front entrance of the facility.

First Aid equipment and materials

Minimum requirements
- Emergency phone numbers and addresses (ambulance, fire, poisons information line). These should be posted on a wall or noticeboard in an obvious position, and perhaps be programmed into the phone memory as well
- Basic First Aid notes or booklet
- Individually wrapped sterile adhesive dressings ($\times$ 50)
- Sterile eye pads
- Sterile coverings for serious wounds
- Triangular bandages
- Safety pins
- Small sterile unmedicated wound dressings
- Medium-sized sterile unmedicated wound dressings
- Large sterile unmedicated wound dressings
- Adhesive tape: 1.25cm wide roll
- Rubber thread or crepe bandages
- Scissors
- Disposable gloves
- Burns module
- Eye-wash module—this kit should be portable
- Resuscitation mask.

Additional recommended items
- Suitable oxygen equipment which must be stored, serviced and used in accordance with well established and rehearsed procedures
- Cotton wool balls (200 g)
- Adhesive dressing strips in assorted sizes, individually sealed packets ($\times$ 100)
- Sterile gauze pieces, 75 mm $\times$ 75 mm
- Adhesive strapping tape, 25 mm
- Liquid skin antiseptic
- Surgical scissors, blunt nose (1 pair)

- Dressing forceps, 125 mm min. (1 pair)
- Kidney tray, stainless steel, 17 cm
- Splinter forceps, tweezers (1 pair)
- Disposable drinking vessels, 200 ml ($\times$ 20)
- Clinical thermometer
- Torch, pocket-size
- Paracetamol tablets, 500 mg ($\times$ 100)
- Soap and nail brush
- Paper towels and dispenser
- Clean garments for use by first-aiders
- Cervical collar
- Ice-packs
- Sunscreen
- Towels.

Any medications should be stored in a separate lockable cupboard, and kept up to date and properly stocked.

Occupational Health and Safety Legislation
All staff should be thoroughly trained in relevant occupational health and safety (OH&S) procedures, including records or report forms that may need to be filled out. Any training should be ongoing, and provide for revision and upgrading of skills and knowledge. Staff should be encouraged to ask for clarification or further information if they are not sure of something relating to OH&S— **'The most dangerous thing of all is ignorance.'** Most Australian State OH&S Acts make provisions for the formation of Health and Safety Committees in the workplace. These can be an excellent way of ensuring that staff are made aware of health and safety issues, and of giving them the opportunity to raise issues of concern relating to OH&S.

Oxygen equipment
If oxygen equipment is available as part of First Aid supplies it should only be used by personnel who have recognised qualifications such as the Royal Life Saving Society Australia (with Oxygen Resuscitation Award or Oxygen Equipment)

Award or the Surf Life Saving Association Advanced Resuscitation Certificate or equivalent standing. Regular refresher or upgrading training is essential for people with such qualifications.

IDENTIFYING HAZARDS

Many exercise facilities have potential, and possibly existing, hazardous situations which should be dealt with immediately. Above all, when exercising (particularly on machines with moving parts), infants and pets should not be allowed into the exercise area.

Regular inspections of a facility can help identify hazards. Ideally the facility should be inspected daily, prior to opening, to ensure that there are no obvious problems. More thorough inspections can be carried out at set intervals, perhaps weekly or monthly. Generally it will be the role of regularly employed staff to carry out such checks. However, casual or sessional staff should be aware of the fact that such checks are carried out, and that any hazardous situations (both existing and potential) of which they are aware, must be reported to the appropriate person.

To aid in regular inspections, devise a safety checklist to ensure that all recognised potential problem areas are checked. Each item can be ticked off to show that it has been checked, and a note or comment made indicating the condition of the item, or any problems noted. Provide spaces on the checklist for the date the inspection was carried out, the name of the person carrying out the inspection, and a signature once the inspection is completed. The checklist can be modified or updated as required to reflect such things as changes in operational procedures, addition of new equipment or facilities, ageing of facilities, and greater awareness of problem areas as a result of previous inspections.

Checklists will vary according to the type of facility being inspected. Ideally an experienced occupational health and safety officer should be involved, in consultation with facility staff, in developing the checklist, advising on any procedures necessary to carrying out a proper inspection, and on methods and procedures for reporting existing or potential hazards.

Sample checklist for safety maintenance in an aerobic facility

When designing a safety checklist, you need to consider every aspect of the workplace, including physical facilities, people involved, materials and equipment, procedures, etc. The safety audit on page 80 is an example of what could be used to check the workplace. Modifications would be needed to suit each individual location, site or workplace.

Using a checklist can help ensure that the safety audit is comprehensive; that you have looked at everything which you had planned to consider; that the checks or audits are standardised so that the same things are looked at each time; and that they are conducted in a logical and efficient order that helps the person(s) carrying out the check achieve the task efficiently and effectively.

PRE-SCREENING CLIENTS

The reason for screening clients is to determine whether their level of health is appropriate for performing the tasks normally done during an exercise routine. This type of procedure can be applied readily to most types of organised physical activity. By assessing the clients you hope to identify high, medium and low risk groups.

Completing suitable screening forms, and obtaining approval from medical doctors where necessary, can reduce the likelihood of legal problems occurring in the future. Ideally advice from an appropriate legal source should be sought regarding the appropriateness and type of screening form to be used.

The following pages provide an example of how a gym might set up its screening processes. The form can be readily modified to suit other physical activities.

BASIC SAFETY AUDIT

Location inspected: .... Date inspected: ....

Code: Tick=good   O=needs upgrading   X=hazardous

Inspected by: ....

No.	Topic	Rating	Remarks
1	**Items to be considered: aerobic room** Room has accessible entry and exit Floor surface in good condition (no splinters, not slippery, floor coverings not lifting or tattered or worn, etc.) Equipment in working condition (stereo free of dust, microphone in working order, mats and steps in good condition, etc.) Mirrors securely fixed, not cracked Stage secure and safe Lighting appropriate and in good condition (e.g. do bulbs need replacing?) [etc.]		
2	**Items to be considered: instructors** Instructors qualified CPR and First Aid updated Someone always available who knows First Aid and CPR Instructors aware of emergency procedures Music original		
3	**Items to be considered: facility** Toilets available and in good condition Male and female showers/change rooms available and in good condition Lockers available and in good condition Parking safe and accessible		
4	**Items to be considered: staff areas** Meeting room for staff Lockers available Toilets/change rooms Security arrangements (e.g. doors lockable)		
5	**Items to be considered: First Aid** Adequate number of First Aid boxes Located in best position Boxes properly stacked and clean Adequate first-aiders (rostered) Names of first-aiders displayed		
6	**Items to be considered: [etc. . . .]**		

SAMPLE SCREENING QUESTIONNAIRE

All information supplied will be treated confidentially.

Name: .... Age: ...... Date of birth: .../.../... Sex: ......

Address: ....

.... Postcode: ....

Phone numbers (home/work): ....

Occupation/employer: ....

Person to be contacted in case of accident: ....

     Phone (w): .... (h) ....

Please place a tick in the space where you are required to answer 'yes', 'no' or 'not sure'

	Yes	No	Not sure
• Have you ever had or do you have a family history of heart disease, stroke, raised cholesterol or sudden death?	...	...	...
• Are you a male over 35 or female over 45 and NOT used to regular exercise?	...	...	...
• Are you on medication or have you been in the last 4 weeks?	...	...	...
• Do you have any infectious diseases or any infections?	...	...	...
• Are you pregnant?	...	...	...
• Have you been hospitalised recently or had any major surgery to any limbs or organs?	...	...	...

Have you had or do you have:

	Yes	No	Not sure
• heart conditions such as stroke, high blood pressure, heart murmur, palpitations, chest pains?	...	...	...
• dizziness or fainting?	...	...	...
• bulimia or anorexia?	...	...	...
• gout, diabetes, epilepsy?	...	...	...
• hernia, ulcers?	...	...	...
• stomach, liver or kidney conditions?	...	...	...
• glandular fever or rheumatic fever?	...	...	...

If you have ticked any of the above, you will be required to take this form plus attached sheet to a doctor for clearance.

Office use only: see attached

Have you ever had or do you have:

	Yes	No	Not sure
• pain in neck, back, knees or ankles?	...	...	...
• arthritis?	...	...	...
• cramps, muscular pain?	...	...	...
• Do you smoke?	...	...	...

• Are you a social drinker? How many drinks per week? What type?   ...   .

• Are you on a diet or have specific allergies? If so, what?   ...   .

If you have ticked any of the above, please ask your instructor for guidance before starting.

Briefly write what type of exercise programs you have performed previously or are doing presently.

....

....

....

....

Aim of exercise program is (please circle):

• weight loss   • weight gain   • muscle gain   • muscle tone   • cardiovascular fitness   • health improvement   • social enjoyment   • sports fitness training   • lower back health   • other

It is recommended that all males over 35 and females over 45 have a Medical Assessment, including an exercise ECG and cholesterol/lipid count.

I recognise that the appraiser is not able to provide me with medical advice with regard to my medical fitness and that this information is used as a guideline to the limitations of my ability to exercise. I have answered the questions to the best of my ability and understand the advice above. I am aware that exercise is not without some risk to the musculoskeletal and cardiorespiratory systems. I hereby certify that I voluntarily participate in exercise at Pecs and Decs Gym and do not hold its organisation or the people in this organisation responsible for, and indemnify them from, any personal loss or damage which may occur as a result of my attendance at Pecs and Decs Gym.

Signed: .... Date: .... Witness: ....

Medical clearance

Dear Doctor,

Your patient, ..., wishes to commence a personal exercise program.

If your patient is taking medication which will affect his/her heart-rate response to exercise, or any other function or system, please indicate manner of effect.

TYPE OF MEDICATION: ....

EFFECT: ....

....

....

Your patient has indicated the following in a pre-exercise health questionnaire:

....

....

....

Please identify any recommendations or restrictions that are appropriate for your patient in this program.

....
....
....

Doctor's name: ....
Clinic, address: ....
Date: .... Phone: (   ) ....
Signature: ....

To be returned to Pecs and Decs Gym, PO Box 777, Abalapac, Qld 4999; Phone (07) 1234 1111

LEGAL LIABILITIES FOR FITNESS INSTRUCTORS

Legal liability has become of increasing significance over recent decades. Recreation professionals, agencies and businesses today may be subject to lawsuits over accidents, provision of inappropriate services, or other aspects such as negligence.

The law relating to negligence is based on precedence from prior legal decisions:

> Negligence is a tort [i.e. a civil wrongdoing], actionable at the suit of a person suffering damage in consequence of the defendant's breach of duty, to take care to refrain from injuring him.
>
> Negligence is the omission to do something, which a reasonable man, guided upon those considerations which ordinarily regulate the conduct of human affairs, would do, or doing something which a prudent and reasonable man would not do. It is simply, neglect of some care which we are bound to exercise toward somebody. Reasonable care must be taken to avoid acts or omissions which can be reasonably foreseen, that would likely cause injury to others.

(*Osborn's Concise Law Dictionary*, 6th edn, ed. J. Bourke.)

A person can only be judged negligent, hence considered liable, if they are considered able to foresee danger. Before a person can be sued for negligence, the following must be determined by the person claiming damages:

a) Legal duty to conform to a standard of behaviour to protect others from unreasonable risk.
b) A breach of that duty caused by failure to conform to the standard required, under the circumstances.
c) A sufficiently close causal connection between the conduct of the individual, and resulting injury to another.
d) Actual injury or loss to the interests of another.

(John Andrews, 'Negligence as it applies to a recreation leader' in *Australian Parks and Recreation Magazine*, Royal Australian Institute of Parks and Recreation.)

Various situations may arise in the recreation industry where negligence and legal liability become an issue. Planners, managers and recreation leaders may all be subject to these concerns. A manager who inappropriately manages a facility or service may be held liable for the results of his actions; a leader who gives incorrect or insufficient leadership may also be held liable.

When is liability a problem?

Liability may become an issue in the following situations:

- Not adhering to established safety standards and procedures when leading a recreation activity
- Proceeding with activities in bad circumstances (e.g. during bad weather, or when equipment is discovered to be faulty)

- Not showing reasonable care (e.g. giving very little attention to someone who has an accident while a lot of attention was given to someone else)
- Condoning or participating in unreasonable risks
- Using dangerous equipment or facilities (e.g. not checking for sharp edges or slippery surfaces in a facility)
- Using dangerous equipment without having adequate skills (e.g. conducting step or weights classes without having the appropriate certification)
- Failing to give proper warnings
- Failing to restrict participation to those who are properly trained or skilled
- Failing to control overcrowding (e.g. letting too many people participate in some activities may raise the risk of accident considerably)
- Failing to become aware of special circumstances (e.g. that a person is diabetic, epileptic or has a heart condition).

CONTRIBUTORY NEGLIGENCE

Contributory negligence occurs where more than one party shares liability for something. Responsibility for care may lie jointly with the recreation leader, the provider of facilities (including equipment), the facility manager, and the person participating in the activity. If a manager and leader make the participant fully aware of all risks involved in an activity, then much of the responsibility for participation is transferred to that person.

Participants then must be aware of the risks to which they are exposing themselves, and must make their own decisions about whether or not to continue with the activity. If there is an accident in such a situation, the participant will be largely liable for their own damages; but depending on circumstances, not necessarily fully liable.

INSURANCE

Liability insurance is available, and increasingly being used by professionals such as consultants, teachers, recreation leaders, fitness instructors and health professionals. One should note that there may be a difference between *liability* and *negligence*, when it comes to insurance policies. Insurance companies may insure a professional against innocent mistakes, but they are unlikely to insure against blatant and premeditated neglect. Even in the safest and most carefully planned situations; accidents can still occur; and they do! An innocent accident resulting in a major lawsuit can destroy the career of a capable but unlucky professional. Proper care together with appropriate insurance policies will save a great deal of heartache for all parties concerned, and perhaps save a career. A relevant industry-based organisation or association should be able to provide you with advice as to what types of insurance policies you might require, and where best to obtain them.

CHAPTER 6

FITNESS TESTING AND ASSESSMENT

Professionals in the health and fitness industry find fitness testing procedures not only useful but a necessity. To see changes and results, pre- and post-testing is essential, whether you wish to improve your fitness, lose weight or run faster. The measures of health and fitness can range from body weight results, anaerobic fitness or elite athlete performance. The goals you wish to achieve need to be measured and monitored.

A simple body-fat test, 12-minute run or sit and reach test can determine a standard which the beginner athlete can attempt to improve on. At the conclusion of a training program, post-test scores are compared to original scores—the results can indicate the level of improvement.

Sometimes it is very useful to complete fitness tests before you begin an exercise program, especially when you are training by yourself and looking for feedback. Working with fitness professionals or personal trainers can provide you with the feedback you require to remain motivated, while individuals training alone can find staying motivated more difficult because positive feedback is harder to come by.

Fitness tests are commonly carried out to:

- Determine a person's maximum aerobic capacity, in order to properly design an appropriate personal exercise program
- Assist with possible detection of any abnormalities, or other risk factors associated with exercise, before embarking on an exercise program
- Evaluate competencies and limitations in muscle, skeletal and nervous systems which might impact on movements undertaken during exercise (e.g. knee injury, flexibility)

- Test body fat levels
- Determine existing body measurements to evaluate later decrease in body fat or increase in muscle
- Determine progressive changes in the various indicators of fitness, such as aerobic capacity, heart-rate, fat levels, flexibility, during and after completion of an exercise program.

All sorts of tests and measurements can be undertaken to gain an indication of a person's fitness. Each has its own purpose, indicating one or several aspects of fitness. One test may not be sufficient for a true indication of the fitness component.

Aerobic fitness can be tested many ways, using a treadmill, bike, rowing machine or similar aerobic fitness equipment. These tests measure the amount of oxygen that can be taken up. There are both submaximal and maximal tests.

Submaximal tests measure the ability to sustain a moderate workload for long periods of time; the subject is exercised at a pre-set level, but not to exhaustion. Examples include the Astrand Bicycle Ergometer, a 12- to 15-minute run, Step test, the Harvard Step Test and the Queen's College Step Test. An individual with a high proportion of slow twitch fibres and a large stroke volume, that is, the volume of each heartbeat, would do well in this type of test.

Health and fitness centres commonly use the cycle ergometer test to place individuals into a fitness category. Advantages of this test are that it is time-efficient, simple and reasonably accurate. The test can, however, favour cyclists, and others who participate in sports where the legs are strongly used, such as runners, while underestimating the fitness of others. Ergometer-style machines that imitate other sports, such as canoeing and rowing, can give a better idea of the fitness of people who participate in those types of sports.

Maximal tests (which measure heart-rate, ECG and recovery) are not important in 'normal' situations, but can have an application with elite athletes. To measure aerobic capacity accurately requires expensive and sophisticated equipment which is often outside the scope of a gymnasium's budget.

WEIGHT

Factors

An individual's weight varies according to:

- Height—taller people are generally heavier
- Bone density
- Percentage body fat
- Diet
- Exercise levels
- Muscle size and mass
- Age
- Sex.

Significance Given that several weight factors, such as height and bone density, tend to change very slowly, any significant change in body weight over a period of a few weeks or months is probably caused by diet, exercise or stress. A change in any of these three factors can readily alter weight.

Variables Time of day, stage of the menstrual cycle, daily food intake and the degree of fluid retention can also affect body weight.

Measurement methods

Scales It is important to weigh yourself (or the person you are testing) under the same conditions every time. For example, with/without shoes, before breakfast, before bed, etc. It is also important to use the same set of scales each time, as there can be considerable variations from one set to another.

Weight in water Special equipment is required for this method, which makes it an expensive technique. However, measuring weight in water is a more accurate method, which can also tell us exactly how much bones, major organs and muscles weigh, compared to body fat percentage.

BLOOD PRESSURE

Blood pressure is a measurement of the resistance of blood against the artery walls. It is stated as a figure like 120/80 mm Hg, which represents the systolic measurement over the diastolic measurement.

Measurement methods Blood pressure measurements should be taken by a qualified fitness trainer or medical practitioner.

Wrap the hollow cuff (an inflated elongated bag that can be fixed around the arm using Velcro) around the left brachial artery (upper arm). Inflate the cuff to restrict blood flow. A stethoscope is held on the inside joint between the upper and lower arm. Slowly release air to reduce pressure. When the first sounds are heard the pressure can be read from a gauge attached to the inflated cuff. This is the systolic pressure. The pressure is further reduced until all sounds stop (meaning blood is flowing freely without causing any vibrations). The pressure is read at this point to give the diastolic pressure.

Factors Depending on an individual's lifestyle and stress levels, a blood pressure reading may differ from the norm.

Significance The diastolic (lower) figure should never be over 90 mm Hg.

The World Health Organisation has defined a reading of systolic 160 mm Hg and diastolic 95 mm Hg as abnormal, requiring treatment and continuing observation.

The National Health Foundation of Australia considers that a person who records a blood pressure reading of 140/90 has borderline hypertension (high blood pressure), and recommends further medical investigation before exercise is continued.

Variables Blood pressure varies considerably throughout the day and night. Variations in posture (sitting, lying, standing), breathing rate, smoking, stress, anxiety, exercise, and caffeine can all raise or lower pressure. These variations can be minimised if the subject is relaxed and does not smoke, exercise or drink tea, coffee or cola, and avoids stress, for at least two hours before blood pressure is taken. Anyone with high blood pressure problems should seek medical advice before commencing an exercise program.

BODY WEIGHT AND PERCENTAGE BODY FAT

The most important information obtained from monitoring the percentage of body fat is determining changes in muscle tissue over time. By determining body fat percentage the mass of the muscles, organs and bone can also be calculated.

Factors

- Diet—quantity and quality
- Exercise—duration, level and frequency of aerobic activities
- Genetics—some people are predisposed to accumulate fat more easily than others.

Men and women go through various stages in their lives when they are more likely to deposit fat. The timing of these fat deposit periods tend to correspond with growth spurts. Growth spurts are, however, very variable due to the individual mixture of genetics, diet and physical activity. Genetic factors determine to a large degree where we deposit fat. Men tend to deposit fat on the abdominal area and women on their thighs, buttocks and hips.

Significance Body fat percentage can be used as a general indicator of health. Remember that it is natural for women to have a higher body fat percentage than men.

Generally acceptable levels of percentage fat for the average female are 17–28 per cent; for the average male 12–21 per cent. Figures for normal, healthy, lean individuals, less than 17

per cent for women, and 12 per cent for men, are not acceptable.

For fit athletes in training, acceptable levels are 12–24 per cent for women, and 7–14 per cent for men. Levels below these figures are generally considered unacceptable, as they can be dangerous, being associated with being associated with poor diet, over-exercising, bulimia, anorexia and/or poor endurance strength.

Some health professionals consider even 12 per cent to be too low a figure for women athletes, while others merely consider it very fit.

A slightly lower percentage of body fat can be acceptable, especially in elite athletes such as triathletes and gymnasts who require minimal body fat.

Variables Percentage body fat figures are influenced by variables such as diet, exercise, accuracy of measurement techniques, and the type of measurement technique used.

Methods of measuring body fat

Skinfold callipers are considered to provide a more accurate measurement of body fat percentage and obesity than height–weight ratio.

Skinfold measurements from multiple sites generally provide a more accurate indication.

For greater accuracy, take three measurements at each site and record the average figure. Sites frequently measured include:

- Abdomen—measure on a vertical fold about 2.5 cm to the right of the navel.
- Calf—measure on the inside right calf at the level of the maximum calf girth.
- Thigh—measure a vertical skinfold midway between the kneecap and the point at which the hip joint bends in the front.
- Triceps—measure a skinfold on the upper arm, mid-way between the shoulder and the elbow.
- Scapula—measure on right side of the body 1.25 cm below the inferior angle of the scapula, following natural lines of the fold.
- Suprailiac—measure a diagonal fold at the front of the hips just above the crest of the ilium.

For very accurate readings use a tape measure,

measuring each site correct to the millimetre. A faint pen mark can be drawn onto the skin to make sure the callipers are in the correct position. Subsequent readings will always be an accurate comparison if this measurement technique is used each time.

The number of sites tested will depend on the method used at the particular fitness centre. The total sum for the calliper reading is converted to body fat percentage utilising a standard table. The subject's gender and age, and the sum of the skinfold reading, are looked up on the table to give the total percentage of body fat.

Many physiology and fitness-testing texts include tables that can be referred to for results. The table you use depends on how many sites were tested. Within your health and fitness centre it is important that you find one table that all the instructors agree with. You may be at a centre that has only a short time available for the entire fitness test so that the fitness team decides to test only two sites. Some tests are more extensive, measuring up to seven or eight sites.

HEIGHT–WEIGHT RATIO

Height needs to be measured with the individual standing bare-footed and erect, with heels flat on the floor. Standard tables suggest the range a person falls into according to their height and weight. For a woman only 160 cm tall and weighing 70 kg, a standard table would categorise her in the overweight range. Ideal weight for this height is said to be about 58 kg. Height–weight ratio is not very accurate, because it does not take into consideration bone density and weight or muscle weight. This person might be an elite bodybuilder or shot-putter. She might have a larger proportion of muscle than the average 160 cm tall woman. Muscle weighs more than fat, therefore such a woman could not really be classified as over-weight or obese. Height–weight tables should be used only as a general guide, and have no real place in a book such as this.

BODY MASS INDEX

Body mass index (BMI) is a frequently used formula for determining obesity:

$$BMI = body\ weight\ (kg) \div height\ (in\ metres)^2$$

(Most of us will need a calculator.)

For example, let us say a man weighs 104 kg and is 183 cm tall. BMI = 104 kg $\div$ 1.83², which gives a BMI of 32. Recommended BMIs fall in the range of 20–25. A BMI of 25–30 is considered to be overweight, and one of 30–39 is considered obese, thus the man in our example is obese.

BMI is generally related to body composition and may also vary due to the sex of the individual. It takes into consideration physiological variables such as height, whether your body frame is large, medium or small, and your body type (i.e. tall and lean, short and muscular). It provides a better estimate of obesity than body weight. It is highly correlated with relative body fat.

HYDROSTATIC (UNDERWATER) WEIGHING

This a method used to calculate body fat percentage from body density. Subjects sit in a chair or sling attached to scales above water level, and the weight in the air is recorded. They are immersed in the water completely (still sitting in the chair attached to the scales); they must fully exhale under water, and their weight is recorded again. This procedure has to be repeated several times until a consistent weight result is obtained. Body density can be calculated using the two figures (weight submerged and weight in air), then the percentage of fat can be calculated from the body density figure. This is based on the principle (discovered by Archimedes) that a body loses an amount of weight under water which is equal to the weight of the water it displaces. Hence, knowing what a given volume of water weighs, it is possible to calculate the volume of a body by using the following formula:

$$BD = M_a \div \left(\frac{M_a - M_w}{D_w} \right) - RV$$

Where: M_a = weight in air
M_w = weight submerged
D_w = density of the water
(this = 1 at 4°C)
RV = residual volume

ELECTRONIC OR LIGHT BODY COMPOSITION ANALYSERS

These are relatively new devices which measure the percentage of body fat by sending a safe near to infra-red light through body tissue. Fat absorbs the light, but lean body tissue reflects it. The device measures the amount of light absorbed relative to the amount reflected, and provides a reading of body fat. This type of device is considered very accurate, and may be used increasingly as it becomes more readily available.

PHYSICAL DIMENSIONS

These are measurements of the physical size of different parts of the body such as height, chest or waist. For example, you might measure changes in waist girth, or chest expansion, or increase in biceps size.

Factors Physical dimensions can change throughout the day due to the effect of gravity; for example, there is more fluid in the legs at the end of the day than in the morning.

Significance Measuring physical dimensions shows not only increase and decrease of measurements, but also overall changes in body shape.

Variables Different people taking measurements can easily result in slight variations in results, as everyone holds a measuring tape a little differently.

Measurement methods

Physical dimension measurements are generally taken with a tape measure.

HEART-RATE

This is the rate at which a person's heart is beating, which is commonly measured at various stages of activity and inactivity for fitness testing. The heart-rate when a person is resting averages around 72 beats per minute (bpm), and is generally a little higher in females than in males. In a very fit person it may be lower. In a very unfit person it may be higher. The heart-rate increases as a result of exercise, in order to deliver more oxygen to the blood and in turn to the muscles.

Factors Heart-rate can vary according to:

- Stress—heart-rate in a person under stress will be higher than average, even if that person is very still.
- Posture—the heart-rate when lying down is lower than when standing or exercising.
- Level of fitness—fitter people have smaller increases in heart-rate in response to increased physical activity; the resting heart-rate is usually lower than average in a fit person (but this is not always the case).
- Activity—with increased activity the heart-rate increases.

Significance The average resting heart-rate is about 72 bpm (beats per minute) for males and 80 bpm for females; rates can differ significantly in trained athletes. Heart-rates can provide a general indication of a person's cardiovascular fitness.

- In a fit person the heart-rate may be as low as 50–65 bpm, while in an unfit person it may be higher then 75 bpm.
- Marathon runners have been known to have a resting heart-rate as low as 35–40 bpm.
- After exercise the heart-rate of a fit person will return to normal faster than in an unfit person. It is possible to get an estimation of fitness by measuring the heart-rate at a standard time (e.g. one, two or five minutes) after exercise.

Measurement methods

These methods can all be self-administered, or performed by the instructor.

Radial pulse (taking the pulse on the wrist): You need a watch with a second hand, or a digital seconds display. Hold the palm of your right hand facing upwards; place the tips of the middle three fingers of the left hand on the wrist joint, below the base of the right thumb, and count the number of beats over six seconds. Multiply this number by ten to give the beats per minute.

Carotid pulse (taking the pulse on the throat): You need a watch with a second hand, or a digital seconds display. Place two fingers (first and second) lightly on the side of the throat, just below the angle of the jaw. You should be able to feel a pulse. Count the number of beats over six seconds. Multiply this number by ten to give the beats per minute.

HEART-RATE MONITORS

In most physical training situations heart-rate monitors are the preferred method for measuring heart-rate, as they give a more accurate measure than manual or 'finger' methods. They have numerous advantages:

- Accuracy—for example, monitors from Polar (a leading brand) have been independently tested as being within 1 beat per minute of electrocardiogram readings at intensities up to 180 bpm.
- They can give continuous, instantaneous readings that can be viewed readily via digital display. This means that the exerciser doesn't have to stop or interrupt an exercise session or evaluation session to perform a manual test. Exercise intensity can be readily adjusted upwards or downwards so that heart-rate remains in the desired training range.
- They are small and light in weight, creating little if any hindrance to carrying out physical activity.
- Some can be programmed to sound an alarm or warning when set heart-rate

ranges are breached, or when set maximum rates are reached.

- They can be used for practically any type of physical activity; waterproofed models are available for activities such as swimming, canoeing and rowing.
- Readings are commonly taken through receptors in a chest strap, which transmit a signal to a watch-type receiver, or to a hand-held receiver monitored by a coach, training partner, or fitness evaluator.

TRAINING ZONE

Training zone refers to a range of the percentage of the maximum heart-rate at which a person trains. Optimally this range is maintained throughout the exercise regime. Training is therefor set at a percentage of the MHR.

> Maximum heart-rate (MHR) is a measure used to determine the peak rate at which the heart should beat when under stress (i.e. being exercised):
>
> $$220 - \text{age (in years)} = \text{MHR}$$
>
> This simple formula is used to determine optimum training intensity.

Different training zones are selected in order to achieve different goals. For example, if you were wanting to work at the minimum level of work-out to achieve fitness you would multiple the MHR by 0.6 (60 per cent). If you wanted to work at a maximum level you would need to multiply the MHR by 0.85 (85 per cent of one's maximum heart-rate).

Example: Sue is a 20-year-old woman who wants to work at a low-impact/moderate pace (i.e. 75 per cent) because she has a foot injury.

$$220 - 20 = 200$$
$$200 \times 0.75 = 150 \text{ bpm}$$

When she takes her pulse for six seconds after warm-up and multiplies it by 10 she should get at least 150 bpm. If the bpm figure is much lower she needs to work harder to achieve her desired work-out level.

Recovery

A fitter individual's heart-rate returns to normal after exercise more quickly than does an unfit individual's heart-rate. Measuring heart-rate 1, 2 and 5 minutes after every exercise session can be a good way to monitor fitness.

After the first week of training an individual might have the following recovery rates:

1 minute: 140 bpm
2 minutes: 130 bpm
5 minutes: 85 bpm

After three months of training comparable figures might be:

1 minute: 143 bpm
2 minutes: 110 bpm
5 minutes: 75 bpm

This demonstrates that after a period of training the heart has become more efficient at recovery. It suggests that the individual has become fitter, but there are no standard figures to prove it. Many factors can affect heart-rate, including heat and high altitude, and must be taken into consideration when assessing the figures. Comparison of heart-rates should not be used to compare individuals with one another, but to monitor an individual over time (self-comparison).

LUNG CAPACITY

Lung volume and capacity change little with training. Vital capacity, which is the amount of air that can be expelled after a maximal inspiration, increases slightly. The residual volume, the air that cannot be moved out of the lungs, shows a slight decrease. These changes are considered to be related. Overall, however, total lung capacity does not change.

The total amount of new air moved into the respiratory passageways each minute is called the respiratory volume. It is measured by the formula:

Respiratory volume (RV) = tidal volume × respiratory rate

Tidal volume is the volume of air inspired or expired per breath. The normal tidal volume of a young adult male is about 500 millilitres and the normal respiratory rate is about 12 breaths per minute, so in this example:

$$RV = 0.5L \times 12$$

which equates to approximately 6 litres per minute.

Factors reducing lung capacity

- Smoking
- Susceptibility to asthma and bronchitis
- Long-term exposure to airborne pollutants (e.g. sawdust, insulation particles, brick dust, coal dust).

Measurement methods

The air that travels in and out of the lungs is measured by a spirometer. This is a drum inverted into a chamber of water, with the drum counterbalanced by a weight. The drum contains a mixture of gases, usually air and oxygen. The subject breathes in and out through a mouth-tube connected to the gas chamber, causing the drum to rise and fall; the degree of rise and fall is measured on a spirogram.

Significance A greater lung capacity enables deeper breathing. Greater amounts of air can be taken into the lungs on each breath, allowing more rapid absorption of oxygen into the body. This enables the muscles to receive oxygen more quickly, making the body switch to the aerobic system more quickly, thus allowing the body to work more efficiently.

Variables affecting measurement With practice, people get better at using a spirometer, breathing out harder and longer, which alters measurements. Respiratory illness can result in decreased measurements.

CARDIOVASCULAR SCORE

The maximum amount of oxygen that a person can utilise per minute is referred to as maximal oxygen uptake (professionally called VO_2max).

This maximum value is sometimes called 'aerobic capacity', which indicates a person's physical fitness. In effect, a person who takes in more oxygen is more likely to have a better functioning heart and lungs, and hence overall cardiovascular fitness.

Factors affecting heart-rate Factors such as caffeine intake, medication, exercise, stress levels, time of day and health at the time of measurement can all affect heart-rate.

Significance Shows how exercise affects heart-rate, and how quickly you recover.

Factors affecting VO$_2$max
- Fitness—regular exercise can improve VO$_2$max by up to 20 per cent
- Blood—blood haemoglobin content can vary between individuals, and in particular between gender (VO$_2$max for females may be up to 30 per cent lower than for males)
- Genetic characteristics
- Type of test—someone who does not exercise regularly will often produce 'better' results on a treadmill than on a cycle ergometer.

Significance Shows the total amount of oxygen that can be utilised by the body.

Variables
- Pulmonary function—abnormal pulmonary function will affect the result
- Muscle twitch fibres—the percentage of muscle twitch fibres in an individual's make-up can limit their maximal oxygen uptake. An individual with a large proportion of slow twitch fibres (red/oxidative) is more likely to be an endurance athlete than a sprinter.
- Cardiovascular limitations caused by age: VO$_2$max decreases by about 10 per cent per decade with ageing, beginning in the late teens for women and mid-twenties for men. This can also be associated with a decrease in cardiorespiratory endurance activity.
- Heart conditions—many people may have to be aware of their limitations to train if they have heart problems.

- Oxygen use—just because muscles can receive more oxygen doesn't mean they can use it; oxygen utilisation depends on the myoglobin content in the muscles and how well it extracts oxygen from the blood.
- Nervous system—the sympathetic nervous stimulates vasodilation and vasoconstriction; vasodilation allows more blood to enter the active skeletal muscles while vasoconstriction occurs in most other tissues and thus assists in diverting blood to the active muscles, together promoting better oxygen delivery around the body.
- Oxidative enzymes—the efficiency of the mitochondria in the cells increases with endurance training.

Measurement methods
The methods of testing aerobic fitness depend on preference and the equipment, time and money available. These tests measure cardiovascular endurance.

VO$_2$MAX TREADMILL TEST

This measures the maximum volume of oxygen which a person can take in over a set period of time (commonly litres of oxygen per minute). This ability to take in and use oxygen varies between individuals. As this test could be dangerous in some situations, *it should be approached with caution* and conducted only by qualified fitness assessors.

Conditions for achieving an accurate reading:

- No eating for one or two hours prior to the test
- No vigorous exercise for at least 24 hours prior
- No smoking for one hour prior
- No caffeinated drinks for at least one hour beforehand
- Patients on blood pressure medication should consult their physician first.

The subject begins exercise at a comfortable

pace, after which exercise intensity increases progressively, usually in one- to three-minute increments, through altering the speed or the incline of the treadmill. This continues until the subject can exercise no longer because of fatigue. At this point the subject may vomit.

During this test the subject breathes through a two-way, lightweight mouthpiece or mask connected to a gas analyser. The oxygen, carbon dioxide and total volume of air breathed are measured throughout the test and the figures used to calculate oxygen consumption. VO_2max is determined by the highest amount of oxygen consumed during exercise, a point usually reached in the final minute of exercise (fatigue).

VO_2max is expressed as a value of litres of oxygen consumed per minute or, when adjusted for body mass, as millilitres of oxygen consumed per kilogram of body mass per minute (ml/kg/min).

BICYCLE ERGOMETER

The equipment for this test is quite inexpensive, accessible and easy to transport. Purchasing a bike with a fitness assessment attachment or purchasing the ergometer separately are the two best ways to assess fitness using a bicycle.

Optional method for assessment

Testing should be carried out on a bike that reads workload based on rpm, with the subject seated at all times on a comfortable seat at the correct height. The leg should be slightly bent when the pedal is at the lowest point of travel.

First get the subject to do a 3-minute warm-up such as walking.

Set the machine at a constant rev (use a low rev range such as 45 rpm).

Ask the subject to ride bike at 45 rpm for at least 3 minutes (sometimes it is best do this over 20 minutes).

Ask the subject to get off bike and sit down.

Take one-minute heart-rate readings after the first minute, second minute and third minute after sitting down (i.e. at one minute

take a reading over one minute; at two minutes take another one-minute reading, and do the same at the third minute). Alternatively, take a 15-second reading then multiply that figure by four to get the beat/minute figure.

Add those three beats-per-minute figures together and divide the total by two.

The resulting figure is known as the Recovery Index. It is used as a heart rate recovery benchmark. It is less technical than VO_2max, but is considered more accurate for estimating recovery.

A satisfactory heart-rate would be in the range 116–128 beats per minute.

FIELD EVALUATION OF CARDIORESPIRATORY ENDURANCE

Most field tests of cardiorespiratory endurance utilise running, jogging, or walking. Studies have aimed at determining how long a person must work to provide accurate results. The physiologist Dr Bruno Balke has demonstrated that an adequate estimate of aerobic capacity is obtainable after as little as 10 minutes of maximal work. Other studies suggest the duration of a running test must be between 10 and 20 minutes to provide a reasonable estimate of aerobic capacity. This is because in shorter runs, of less than eight to 10 minutes, much of the energy used comes from anaerobic sources.

As the duration of a 'best-effort' run increases, the demand on the anaerobic energy component is less, decreasing to less than 10 per cent after 10 minutes. The significant point is that if maximum work is performed for 10–20 minutes, the predominant energy source is dependent on the utilisation of oxygen; thus an adequate estimate of the subject's aerobic capacity will result.

Five fitness classifications are provided in Tables 1 and 2 to assist in rating fitness according to the time required for women to run 2.4 km or men 3.2 km. In addition, because the time

Table 1: Classification of 2.4 km run times for young adult females

Fitness category	Time in minutes	Estimated maximal oxygen uptake equivalents
Super	Faster than 11:30	50 ml/kg min or higher
Excellent	11:30 to 12:59	49.9 to 44.0 ml/kg min
Good	13:00 to 14:29	43.9 to 38.0 ml/kg min
Fair	14:30 to 15:59	37.9 to 32.0 ml/kg min
Poor	16:00 or slower	31.9 ml/kg min or lower

Table 2: Classification of 3.2 km run times for young adult males

Fitness category	Time in minutes	Estimated maximal oxygen uptake equivalents
Super	Faster than 12:00	55 ml/kg min or higher
Excellent	12:00 to 13:59	54.9 to 50 ml/kg min
Good	14:00 to 15:59	49.9 to 45 ml/kg min
Fair	16:00 to 17:59	44.9 to 40 ml/kg min
Poor	18:00 or slower	39.9 ml/kg or slower

to run these distances correlates very well with maximal oxygen uptake, estimates of aerobic capacity are given in accordance with running times.

12-MINUTE FITNESS TEST

Cardiorespiratory fitness can be gauged very easily by this test.

1. Find an oval or some other circuit you can run around. Measure the distance of the course you intend to run (a sportsground might be 250 metres around the boundary, for instance). This can be measured in approximate terms by pacing out the circuit.
2. Keeping track of the time, run around the course as many times as you are able to in 12 minutes. Use effort, but don't kill yourself. You should be puffing away at the end of 12 minutes.
3. Multiply the number of laps by the distance of the circuit to calculate the total distance run.
4. Compare your performance with figures in

the following table which show cardiorespiratory fitness levels for different levels of performance.

Distance run	Result for young adult women	Result for young adult men
3800 m	Super-human	Super-fit
2800 m	Super-fit	Excellent
2600 m	Excellent	Good
2300 m	Good	Fair
2000 m	Fair	Poor
1500 m	Poor	Very poor

Before any fitness test

Before conducting any fitness test, the client should always be asked a series of questions concerning their health. This is because their current status of health (on the day of the test, as well as previously) can impact on both the safety and reliability of the test. For example, the fitness of a person suffering from hay fever or a sore neck on the day of the test will not be properly reflected by the test; also it might be unwise for an unwell person to undertake the exercises involved in the testing procedure.

Questions which must be asked:

- Have you ever been diagnosed with a heart or lung condition and advised to be careful about exercise?
- Do you have a tendency to faint?
- Have you experienced abnormal chest pain or dizziness in the past month? If so, do you have medical clearance to exercise? See Chapter 5.
- Are you suffering any infection or illness at present?
- Are you taking any medication, or has medication been recommended?
- Do you have any muscular, bone or joint problem which is sometimes aggravated by exercise?
- Do you smoke?

Note: If any *yes* replies are given, ensure a medical clearance is obtained.

Test conditions

Ideal conditions for conducting a fitness test:

- Air temperature between 18 and 20°C
- Ample ventilation (air movement, but not strong, distracting winds)
- The subject should not smoke or be exposed to polluted air or smoke within two hours of testing
- The subject should not be suffering any infections (e.g. cold. flu)
- The subject should ideally have not eaten for two hours prior to the test
- The subject should have not exercised or undertaken heavy work within two hours of the test.

What combination of tests?

The big decisions in any fitness assessment are: What tests should be run? What tests should be left out? Running too many tests can become tedious, time-consuming and costly for both trainer/fitness centre and the client. If too few tests are conducted, you will not get a proper indication of the subject's fitness components.

Before deciding which tests to conduct, you need to determine:

- How much time should be allowed to do the tests (between 30 and 60 minutes)
- What aspects of the person's fitness are most critical—ask is it fitness, strength, flexibility?
- How precise do the results need to be—is a general indication of fitness sufficient? In the case of a professional athlete a precise measurement may be required.

Further reading on fitness testing

Bosco, J.S. and Gustafson, W.F. (1983), *Measurement and Evaluation in Physical Education, Fitness and Sports*, Prentice Hall, New Jersey

Hastad, D.N. and Lacy, A.C. (1994), *Measurement and Evaluation in Physical Education and Exercise*, 2nd edn, Gorsuch Scarisbrick, Arizona

Jones, K. and Barker, K. (1996), *Human Movement Explained*, Butterworth-Heinemann, Oxford

CHAPTER 7

PROGRAMMING, MOTIVATION AND LEADERSHIP

MANAGING EXERCISE PROGRAMS

An exercise program consists of one or several sequences of training units, each sequence being carried out during a single training session.

Exercise unit = a single type of activity, or a single well-defined task.
Example: Walking 1 km or lifting a specified weight in a certain way for 10 repetitions.

Exercise segment = a combination of similar training units.
Example: A series of different aerobic exercises, or a series of different stretching exercises.

Exercise session = a combination of training segments, undertaken as a sequence at the same point in time.
Example: An aerobic segment followed by a stretching segment followed by a segment of weights (i.e. resistance training).

Exercise program = a schedule for undertaking exercise sessions.
Example: This typically involves at least three exercise sessions per week. It may involve more. The exercise sessions may all be the same, or different types of exercise sessions may be undertaken at different points during the program.

A person's individual capacity to undertake exercise depends upon age, sex and level of fitness. The amount of energy used for all exercise segments together, in a training session, is called the *overload* (also called training stimulus). Different people, the fit and the unfit, will have different capacities to undertake the same exercise program, thus the impact of the same program on different individuals will vary. This variation is called the *strain*. The way a person's strain impacts upon the exercise undertaken is called the *training stress*.

FITNESS/AEROBICS CLASS DESIGN

Fitness and aerobic classes commonly have warm-up, cardiovascular conditioning, resistance conditioning and cool-down components, requiring a qualified professional instructor to design and conduct them.

Class intensity and duration

How is this determined? The type of class timetabled at the health and fitness centre will depend on the clients' goals. Sessions catering for clients who want primarily to gain cardiovascular fitness will need to have at least 20 minutes in the cardiovascular phase. The longer this phase the fitter the participants will become. Keeping in mind that classes are commonly one hour in duration, and include warm-up and resistance/cool-down components which can take up 20 or 30 minutes, then realistically it must be said that a one-hour aerobic class will provide participants with only a limited fitness component.

If the duration of the class is set, the other factor to consider is intensity. The level of fitness gained will depend on how hard the participant works. The target for increasing fitness is at least 60 per cent of the participant's maximum heart-rate. Exercisers who work at 75 per cent MHR or more will become noticeably fitter. The maximum rate at which participants should work is 85 per cent MHR. Above this and they are working in the anaerobic stage, which cannot be continued for very long due to lactic acid build-up and fatigue.

PRE-CLASS SCREENING

Before beginners start an exercise class it is important that instructors and staff know their goals, fitness level and medical history/condition. With 30 people in a class, one instructor cannot monitor participants individually. Any medical concerns therefore must be raised beforehand. Someone who wants to build strength, for example, and does not care about cardiovascular endurance, will not be suited by an advanced fitness class which goes for 90 minutes. Pre-class screening (see pages 81–2) can help the instructor or gym staff advise participants which class will best suit their needs.

INTRODUCTION

Before the class begins the instructor should:

- Make an introduction to the class
- Welcome everyone, especially new members
- Ask for questions
- Provide any necessary instructions (e.g. location of toilets, water fountain).

People who are new need to have explained to them what to expect, what to do if they cannot keep up, and asked if they have any questions. Sometimes it is better to find out first exactly who is new to aerobics and brief them before you introduce yourself to the remainder of the class. People with injuries need to know what precautions to take and you need to ensure they have seen a medical practitioner before joining the class.

INTRA-CLASS INSTRUCTION

During the class participants need plenty of clear, concise instruction. A good aerobics instructor provides motivation and verbal cues for what is coming up, and does not babble on all the time. If too much information is being given participants may get 'lost' within an activity or sequence, or worse, tune out. This can lead to falling levels of motivation and rising numbers of accidents, as class members bump into each other or use incorrect technique.

Too many instructors get caught up in chatting about their weekend, often in an effort to create a friendly atmosphere, which unfortunately comes out a muffled mess. Think of the following points for your next class:

- **Countdown** Always count the next move in unless it is really obvious. Towards the conclusion of the class the next move may be known because you have already spent 20 to 30 minutes practising it.
- **Motivation** Provide both verbal and non-verbal cues (smiles, nods and winks) to generate excitement with clients. Make this sound different each time, because it is motivation you are providing, not a tape recording. Even 'good job' repeated too often, in no matter how many different tones, gets boring.
- **Be concise** Choose what you want to say carefully and say it without adding unnecessary information. Do not get lost with what you are trying to get across. Is it technique, motivation, counting down or encouragement? Choose your words and make them quick, clear and concise.
- **Heart monitoring** During the class heart-rate should be monitored, especially in people wanting to increase fitness. Resting (before the class), active (during the class) and post-exercise (after the class) heart-rates

should ideally be taken by each participant. This is extremely important for individuals with any type of heart/medical problems.

- **Choreography** The class must be pitched carefully at the type of clients attending. A complex dance routine may be too hard for people just trying to get fit, for those with little experience of such classes, or for those with poor coordination. They will spend most of their time just trying to keep up with the sequence of movements. In the end they will leave the class because their goals are not being achieved.

PROGRAMMING AN EXERCISE SESSION

Programming simply means planning an exercise session (or activity) before you do it. Programming should be second nature for a fitness instructor. If you are working alone to get fit, programming will allow you to collect your thoughts and focus on what you need to achieve through exercise.

Why do we have a program in the first place?

A written program gives the instructor a step-by-step guide to what should be taking place, including the correct order and type of activities to be carried out to reduce the likelihood of injuries, soreness, and to achieve the desired benefits. It enables the instructor to best fit activities into a set timeframe. It can be used as a promotional tool when you describe to potential participants the activities they will be involved in.

A written program can also be used as a record to chart progress over time; as trends and fitness levels change so will successive programs. It could also be an important record in case of legal action against the facility or instructor for such things as injuries incurred as a result of an aerobic fitness class. It is recommended that programs/lesson plans be kept for 10 years in case of a claim.

Be systematic and write everything down!

The proper way to develop a program is a step-by-step process, in which you write down what you decide at each stage.

DESIGNING AN EXERCISE PROGRAM

An exercise program should be designed to motivate participants to come to a class and to stay involved. In physical terms it should be designed to ease participants in and out of a period of higher heart-rate without causing a level of stress or discomfort that could be dangerous and/or discourage participants from returning to future exercise sessions.

1. DECIDE WHO THE PROGRAM IS BEING DESIGNED FOR

Is it for yourself alone? Perhaps for you and a small group of friends? Perhaps for an exercise class which you are going to lead? You need to have some knowledge of the other participants. If they don't exercise regularly already, it is generally wise to carry out a fitness test before settling on too many details. This enables you to plan a program which best fits the participants' capabilities. (See Sample Screening Questionnaire Checklist on page 81–3.)

2. DECIDE ON THE AIM OF THE PROGRAM

Any program should have a warm-up and cool-down phase, but the main body might aim to achieve any combination of the following:

Improving/maintaining cardiorespiratory fitness

To achieve this participants need ideally to keep their heart-rate between 70 and 85 per cent of their maximum heart-rate for at least 20 minutes of the class. The longer the heart-rate remains this high the more the individual is increasing their fitness.

People who do not exercise regularly should start with a training heart-rate (THR) of 60 per cent of the maximum heart-rate (MHR) for their age group, exercising a minimum of three times per week. For people of medium fitness who are trying to increase or maintain reasonable fitness a THR of 60–75 per cent is appropriate for 20–60 minutes per session, exercising in three or four sessions a week. For athletes, reaching a THR of 70–85 per cent five times or more per week, for up to one hour each time, is appropriate.

To calculate maximum heart-rate and how to work at 70–85 per cent of this utilise the formula:

$$220 - \text{age in years} = \text{maximum heart-rate}$$

Multiply this figure by both 0.7 and 0.85 to get the target heart-rate range.

Example: 25-year-old person:

$$220 - 25 = 195$$
$$195 \times 0.7 = 136, \text{ and}$$
$$195 \times 0.85 = 165$$

This individual needs to work between 136 and 165 beats per minute to achieve a suitable cardiorespiratory training effect.

The heart-rate measured at the radial or carotid pulse should fall between 135 and 165 for the 25-year-old to achieve the required training effect. If the measurement is outside the range the participant needs to either work harder or slow down. Working above 85 per cent (more than 165 bpm) is achieving results in the anaerobic fitness component and needs to work at a lesser intensity; working below this range (less than 135 bpm) means increased intensity is required (bigger, faster or higher impact movements) to achieve optimum results.

Building strength in specific muscles

Increasing strength in major muscle groups can be done through designing work-outs specific to that particular group. Let us say the legs are to be toned and strength increased—an appropriate series of leg exercises needs to be performed, including squats, isolation thigh and gluteal work and general aerobics jogging (impact).

Building general muscular strength

Work-outs can be designed to give the entire body a complete work-out, therefore increasing overall muscular strength. This can be achieved through big movements of the entire body with large leg and arm actions.

Improving flexibility

This can be achieved primarily in the beginning and the conclusion of the class. After the participants have warmed up they should perform a series of stretches to decrease the risk of injury. These exercises can also be very effective in increasing flexibility. Stretches need to be held for at least 20–30 seconds and often repeated. Some stretches may be performed with the assistance of another person to increase the resistance applied. If flexibility is to be one of the aims of the fitness class then more muscle groups will need to be stretched, the stretches will need to be held for longer and more than one repetition will need to be performed. Stretch classes are becoming very popular in aerobic timetables because of increasing concern, especially among the elderly, about poor mobility.

Stretches need to be specific to the particular muscle group that is being exercised. For example, an intense leg work-out could be followed by a series of gluteal, hip flexor, quadriceps, hamstring and calf-muscle stretches.

Relaxation

The final component of an exercise class is the cool-down, where often a relaxation section may be included. This can take from five to 15 minutes depending on the type of class and the time available. Some classes, often referred to as yoga or meditation classes, may have 45–60 minutes of just relaxation/stretching exercises. This is a great way to take time out. Such classes are definitely not aerobics-based, but are still considered a form of aerobics, on the aerobic timetable, in gyms and health clubs.

3. DURATION OF SESSIONS

The duration and frequency of sessions will depend on what you are trying to achieve. This might be influenced by both the aim/s of the program and the time available (some people have limited time to exercise). A session for maintenance of reasonable cardiorespiratory fitness might be as little as 30 minutes three times a week. A session targeting a number of other specific benefits might be as much as one hour or even longer.

4. WRITE DOWN WHAT SHOULD BE DONE WITHIN A TIMED FRAMEWORK

This covers what you are going to do and how long you are going to spend on each component/exercise. You might also include a list of equipment required.

5. REVIEW

Any program should be continually reviewed. The longer people participate in a class, the more their abilities and fitness levels should change; the program they are undertaking should change to suit. This review might involve routine fitness testing, and adjusting the type, difficulty or intensity of exercises accordingly.

A TYPICAL AEROBICS CLASS

1. Introduction/welcome
2. The warm-up stage
3. The main body of exercise—what will be specifically focused on during this session?
4. Conclusion.

INTRODUCTION/WELCOME

- This is the time to introduce yourself to participants you have not already met, and to welcome everyone to the class. This can be a very important step in encouraging and involving participants. A little personal attention at this stage can really make a new class member feel as though they belong

and are welcome. New members may feel nervous or apprehensive about attending in the first place and this will help break the barrier.
- Check off class rolls—or check that everyone has paid!
- This is also a good time to check if any participants have any problems they might want to raise (e.g. need to leave early, have a sore back or other muscle soreness after the last session, want to buy certain equipment from you or the facility, etc.). Some of these problems may need to be deferred until after the class has been run to minimise loss of class time, but they should at least be acknowledged.
- A brief description of what the class is going to do can help prepare participants mentally and ensure a smoother passage from one type of activity to the next.
- Instructions can also be given about the use of equipment at this stage, rather than stopping and explaining during the exercise session, which reduces the session's effectiveness.
- The introduction is a good chance to 'feel out' the mood of class members and expose them to the positive environment created by your motivation and cheerful personality.

Configurations or patterns for movement:
- Arrange everyone in one or several lines, facing the instructor
- Arrange one line to follow the leader in a circle
- Allow people to take positions at random (if there is sufficient room)
- Arrange participants in a circle with the instructor in the middle.

WARM-UP STAGE

Participants are more susceptible to muscle tissue injuries, damage to their joints and cardiac problems if they exercise without warming up first for at least 10 minutes. Warming up does the following:

- It gets the muscles moving and in doing so begins to lubricate the joints.
- It gently stretches the muscles, conditioning them for more vigorous movements to follow.
- It increases the heart-rate and respiration slowly, which is safer than a rapid increase.
- It gradually increases the thermal temperature of tissues which may be cold when exercise commences. This increased temperature increases blood flow, increases the capacity to take in and utilise oxygen (i.e. improves VO_2max), and helps the transmission of impulses through the nerves.
- The hormone system is alerted.
- Energy sources become activated.
- It increases activity in the central nervous system, which leads to faster reaction times.
- It prepares the class psychologically for more vigorous exercise.

This warm-up can be achieved by any gentle movement such as walking, gradually increasing the intensity or effort, and ensuring that a wide variety of muscles in all parts of the body are moving.

There are five aspects to the warm-up:

- The overall body temperature is increased by overall general movement such as walking and low-impact aerobic movements. The heart-rate should be increased gradually and sustained at a raised level for perhaps five minutes. The intensity and duration of this part of the exercise will depend upon the individual's level of fitness and the environmental conditions.
- Major muscle groups should be utilised first, then smaller groups.
- Blood flow to specific areas may need to be increased during warm-up. The muscles targeted, and the importance of this, will depend on the condition of the individual and the purpose of the exercise session. For example, if exercise is being undertaken as therapy for an arm injury, then prescribed arm exercises might be important during this stage.
- The muscles to be targeted in the exercise session should be stretched gradually. The range of exercises prescribed in this warm-up stage should encompass comfortable stretches, each of at least 20 seconds duration.
- The joints which are to be involved in the exercise session should be moved gently at first, with the intensity and range of movement gradually increasing.

1. The aerobic warm-up stage

This stage should aim to gradually increase heart-rate and respiration, thus minimising any stress placed on the heart. A participant should not be puffing hard at the end of the warm-up. This stage, which should take 8–10 minutes, has been performed correctly if the person is breathing more deeply and the heart is pumping faster, but they are still not out of breath.

Appropriate movements for this stage are:

- Low-impact movements with one foot always in contact with the ground
- Simple movements with no turning/ pivoting
- Short and easy-to-remember sequences/ combinations facing the front.

If the aerobic warm-up in a typical exercise to music session is fast, high impact and turns towards the back of the room, the participants risk getting injured and also tend to get lost with what they are doing. The first 10 minutes needs to be easy to follow, allowing time to psychologically prepare for what is coming up.

2. The pre-stretch stage

This phase of stretching aims to fully loosen muscles to achieve the maximum range of motion. If the muscles and joints are not fully warmed up first, stretching may not prevent injury to the muscles. Never try to extend or contract muscles fully while still feeling cold or, even worse, shivering. Do not try to fully extend muscles in a stretch if the muscles are still feeling tight. Do not bounce while stretching, as this can cause tearing of tissues. Each stretch should be held for a minimum of 20–30 seconds.

It is appropriate to do 4–6 types of stretches in this stage which should work on all of the muscles to be used in the class. A good selection might include a calf stretch, hamstring stretch, quadriceps stretch, hip flexor stretch, pectoral stretch and shoulder/deltoid stretch.

MAIN BODY OF THE EXERCISE SESSION

This is the part of the exercise session which takes the longest time and contributes the most towards the overall fitness of the participant. It should be planned according to the goals of the participants. If the warm-up section has been conducted properly, by this time the muscles and joints should be adequately warmed up, and able to withstand optimum levels of exercise within appropriate limits for the individual concerned. Even though the muscles and joints might be capable of optimum movement during this stage, however, the participant's energy systems are probably not capable of maintaining optimum movement throughout the whole of this part of the exercise session.

Sustained movement at 60 per cent or more of the individual's maximum heart-rate, or medium intensity exercise, will utilise the source carbohydrate in the body, which after a certain period will move on to using fats as its main source of energy. The terms 'sustained' or 'excessive' movement, 'medium' or 'high' activity, etc., are relative, meaning different things to different people according to their levels of fitness and strength. Excessive movement at a high intensity may derive energy from body tissues, which can be dangerous and, in a worst-case scenario, actually cause destruction of muscle tissues.

Generally, this part of the session should be designed to incorporate periods of high intensity (but not excessive) movement interspersed with periods of sustained aerobic activity at a medium level of intensity.

A sequence of different activities should be programmed throughout this session, each one utilising different muscle groups from the previous exercise. Doing this will reduce the chance of muscle fatigue, and allow muscles to replenish stores of energy ready for the next period utilising the same muscle group. The duration of this stage may be as little as 20 minutes or up to 45 minutes or longer. At longer durations it becomes increasingly important to manage the intensity of exercise carefully to ensure a useful but safe level of exertion.

The number of different exercises incorporated into this stage will vary according to what is desired from the exercise session. The same type of exercise, or variations of it, might or might not be repeated several times. The amount of each exercise will vary according to the participant's level of fitness and the intensity with which the exercise is being performed.

In many classes, performance capacity will vary greatly from person to person. In order to make a program plan relevant to different people of differing capacities, the different exercises must be graded in terms of quantity and intensity.

- The level of intensity can be planned as a percentage of the individuals' optimum capacity—for example, they could be told to work at 80 per cent of optimum capacity.
- The exercise can be programmed either as a time (duration) or as a quantity (number)—for example, the class could be told to do star jumps for two minutes, or to do 20 star jumps then go to a medium-paced jogging on the spot.

Structured routine

A typical structured sequence for part of this stage of an aerobics class, depending on the type of class, instructor and participants, would be:

step touch forwards × 4
grapevine backwards × 2
flick kick × 4
side taps × 4

(Please refer to figures on pages 103 and 104 for grapevine and side tap movements.)

This takes 32 counts and is a simple block of choreography that travels forwards and backwards and includes high- and low-impact movements.

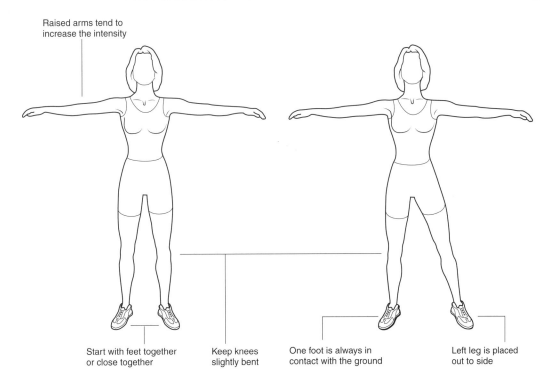

Raised arms tend to increase the intensity

Start with feet together or close together

Keep knees slightly bent

One foot is always in contact with the ground

Left leg is placed out to side

STEP GRAPEVINE

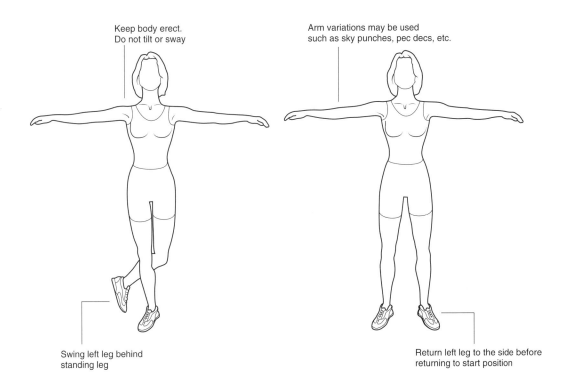

Keep body erect. Do not tilt or sway

Arm variations may be used such as sky punches, pec decs, etc.

Swing left leg behind standing leg

Return left leg to the side before returning to start position

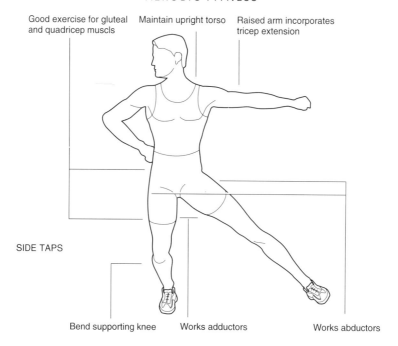

Good exercise for gluteal and quadricep muscls

Maintain uprigcht torso

Raised arm incorporates tricep extension

SIDE TAPS

Bend supporting knee   Works adductors   Works abductors

Such routines can be put together to keep the class thinking, motivated and working hard.

Simple routine

Some classes may not like structured or choreo-graphed routines. This preference can be catered for in a simpler format, with small movements/sequences added on one after the other. An example of this would be:

grapevines × 32 counts
walk forwards and backwards × 32 counts
alternating step knee × 32 counts, etc.

(See the figure opposite for alternating step knee movement.)

These movements performed in blocks of 32 counts allow participants time to practise and master the moves. Numerous movements can be used in this way in this section; it is up to the instructor to gauge what the class wants and what it is ready for.

RECOVERY

During vigorous exercise, the heart pumps fast, body temperature increases and the normal cooling mechanism of sweating comes into play. Recovery is important in classes where hard

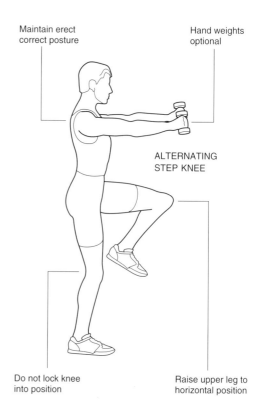

Maintain erect correct posture

Hand weights optional

ALTERNATING STEP KNEE

Do not lock knee into position

Raise upper leg to horizontal position

work-outs are performed on the muscles. A weights or body-sculpt class may have the legs performing squats and lunges for a few minutes at a time—after this the legs require a rest. The next movement could thus be an upper body action, or light walking around the room. For example, work the legs, walk around the room, work the biceps, work the shoulders, and so on, providing particular muscle groups with a recovery period which allows lactic acid to be removed and tension to be released.

In a high-intensity aerobics class, however, recovery should be left until the cool-down section, allowing maximum intensity and duration of continuous work-out.

Muscle conditioning during the class

Muscle condition can be improved to do either or both of the following:

- Move against greater weights or forces—if a muscle can move a greater force it is said to have greater strength
- Move for a longer period of time before tiring—if a muscle can work for longer it is said to have greater endurance, which is the same as greater muscle tone.

The type of exercise required here involves carrying repetitions of the same exercise in a sequence. Each exercise aims to work a particular muscle or group of muscles in a way that is safe, without straining or tearing, but which provides a resistance that challenges that muscle.

The three variables in this type of exercise are:

1. The muscle or combination of muscles being worked
2. The amount of force being pitched against the muscle
3. The number of repetitions.

A typical sequence will involve exercising the following groups of muscles one after the other: legs, shoulders, biceps, triceps, chest, back, abdominals, buttocks and hips.

- Try to isolate the muscles you wish to

develop, using those muscles as much as possible and other muscles as little as possible.
- Have a definite start and finish to each repetition—repetitions should not flow into each other, nor should there be a break between them.
- Bouncing or rapid movements will reduce the muscle-toning effect.
- Never do toning exercises unless the body is first warmed up.

The number of exercises included in this section will depend upon what you are trying to achieve. If the aim is to achieve a general all-round conditioning of main muscle groups, you may choose to incorporate around six different exercises, each dealing with different muscles. If the aim is more targeted—for example, a sports person wishing to develop specific muscles used in their sport— the number of exercises will be determined by the specific muscles being targeted. A set of four to five exercises per muscle group might be performed. Exercises may include push-ups, back arches and abdominal work.

The format suggested here for concluding the session will provide a five to 10 minute muscle-conditioning stage.

CONCLUDING THE EXERCISE SESSION

There are three stages which can be worked through at the end of an exercise session—a cool-down stage, a muscle-conditioning stage within the cool-down, and a stretching stage.

Cool-down stage

Muscles, heart and lungs are returned to their normal condition. If this is done correctly, there is much less chance of any negative after affects or injury; including heart stress, or general soreness.

Muscle-conditioning stage during the cool-down

This stage is not essential. Its inclusion depends on available time and the type of class being conducted. The advantage of undertaking muscle-toning exercises at this point in an exercise session is that the muscles are still warm and in an ideal condition to work on building muscle strength through resistance exercises. It is also a great way to cool the body slowly and decrease the heart-rate towards normal before concluding the class.

Push-ups Come down slowly to the knees and place the hands on the floor. Level 1 can be performed on the knees and hands with the bottom in the air. The chest is taken towards the ground, keeping the abdominals tight. In level 2 the body is straighter but the participant is still on the knees. Level 3 is performed with the toes on the floor. Repetitions of 8 should be performed, with 3 or 4 sets. Emphasise that participants must work at only that level which they are capable of and perfect it before moving up to the next level—perhaps at the next class.

Back arches Excellent for strengthening lower back muscles, especially where abdominal work is always completed fully, when back muscles may be underworked. Take a position face down with one hand under the forehead. The other arm and the opposite leg are raised, keeping the hips on the ground. This is performed slowly, with control, and the back muscles should be squeezed. Continue for 8–10 repetitions, then swap to the other side.

An alternative exercise is done with both hands under the chin and the upper body lifting into the air. This again is performed with control.

Abdominal work When performing abdominal work it is extremely important that participants master the correct technique. The hands should be clasped together and placed behind the head to support the neck. The eyes are towards the roof and the head is held in a neutral position. Lift the upper body until the shoulder-blades are just off the ground. Avoid lifting the upper body higher than halfway, when the hip flexors come into action. Hip flexors that are too tight can create problems with the lower back that you are trying to avoid.

Rotating movements working the oblique muscles can be performed at different rhythms to provide variety—for example, 2 counts up and 2 counts down, or curling up and pulsing the upper body on the spot before returning to the ground.

Stretching stage

Though not an essential stage, stretching does help maintain flexibility and can help reduce any muscle soreness after exercise. This stage should take three to five minutes to complete, and should stretch all of the same muscles that were used during the exercise session.

The whole cool-down stage should take at least five minutes, and preferably eight to 10 minutes. The longer the stretch phase the better. It is very important to remind class members at this point why they are doing an activity/ stretch and of the importance of doing a cool-down after their session. This stage is a great time to educate and build rapport with members of your class. Some participants may think that the main part of the session is over and that it is okay to slip out early, but this is a very important stage to decrease the chance of injuries and muscle soreness. The cool-down is vital, and relates to their overall training results.

- The music could be turned down to make giving directions easier
- Cool-down movements should use muscles fully, in long gentle movements decreasing in vigour, *not* short jerky movements that do not fully extend the muscles
- Keep moving at all times during the cool-down, slowing gradually; do not go from intense exercise to mild, to a 30-second stop, and then return to slow exercise
- The cool-down aids in the removal of wastes that may have built up in the muscles
- Use similar exercises to those used in the initial warm-up stage.
- *Do not skip the cool-down stage.*

WRITING AN EXERCISE PROGRAM

You might construct an exercise program under the following headings, and set it out as in the example on page 108.

1. Name of program
2. Date, time and location of class (if relevant)
3. Method of delivery, e.g. from the water, out of the water (for an aqua-erobics class), with PA system or without, and so on
4. Aims and objectives, including introductory comments, topics to be addressed with class members
5. Warm-up phase, listing duration and sequencing of the parts
6. Main body of exercise, listing duration and sequencing of the parts
7. Cool-down phase, listing duration and sequencing of the parts
8. References—any books or other sources to be consulted in preparation
9. Facilities, materials and equipment—list any requirements for the program.

Devising relevant sets of exercises

No movement in an aerobics routine should be repeated too many times, especially if the same leg is leading. Movements should be mixed up to provide variety. Several high-impact moves in a row may be too difficult for some people to continue with, so provide a low-impact option or mix the moves.

With muscle-conditioning exercises, three or four sets are appropriate on any one muscle group. Work larger muscle groups before moving onto smaller muscle groups.

TYPES OF CLASSES

Aerobics classes take on many different types and formats depending on the health and fitness centre you work at or attend. You may come across:

- Hi Impact Aerobics—movements with both feet off the ground at the same time
- Lo Impact Aerobics—movements with at least one foot in contact with the ground at all times
- Hi-Lo Impact Aerobics—a mix of both high- and low-impact aerobics.
- Step—a low- or high-impact class utilising a step/platform to step up and down on
- Advanced—high impact, very choreographed movements and combinations, or a fast fitness class incorporating lots of running
- Moderate Pace—hi-lo class
- Beginners—low impact
- Body Sculpt—a class utilising weights and muscle-conditioning work, beginning with a warm-up and maybe including a cardiovascular section; also called body blitz, tummy, hips and thighs (THT), toning class
- Pump/Power Bar—an exercise to music class using a barbell to complete a weight work-out covering all major muscle groups
- Interval—a mixture of hi-lo aerobics and weights; it may consist of 10 minutes aerobics, 5 minutes weights, etc.
- Tri—combined step, aerobics and weights.

You will find similar classes under many different names, but wherever you go the same types of classes will be offered. It is up to you to find which one you prefer and enjoy participating in.

SPECIAL CATEGORY CLASSES
Mature/older adults

This group can make up a great proportion of your clientele. They generally do not like loud music, so keep it soft or at a medium level. Most prefer low-key surroundings, so avoid bright lights, mirrors, posters of super-fit young people. Older participants are often more concerned about joint movement and flexibility than weight loss and can relate better to an older instructor who shows respect and individual attention to their requirements. Many people in this group attend for social reasons, to meet others and relax.

NAME OF PROGRAM: .... DATE: .... LOCATION: ....

TIME OF CLASS: .... TIME ALLOCATED FOR CLASS: ....

METHOD OF DELIVERY: .... REFERENCES: ....

EQUIPMENT: ....

SESSION OBJECTIVES: .... TEACHING POINTS: .... EVALUATION: ....

DIAGRAMS/TIME ALLOCATED: ....

WARM-UP/STRETCHES: ....

MAIN BODY: ....

COOL-DOWN: ....

CONDITIONING PHASE: ....

STRETCHING PHASE: ....

Professional athletes/competitive sportspeople

This can be a hard group to cater for because its members vary considerably in the type of sports they are involved in, and elite athletes may require very specialised fitness components. The triathlete, swimmer, runner or aerobics-orientated person will want a hard, advanced class to challenge their fitness. The type of training employed will depend on the type of sport and the fitness components to be improved. You may find elite athletes require personal training, one-on-one, to best achieve their goals.

Personal training is becoming more and more popular, but is expensive and so limited to those who can afford it. It is a great way, however, to increase motivation and improve knowledge and technique. Personal trainers need to have up-to-date knowledge of the latest techniques and research in the fitness industry.

Beginners

Beginners are usually a little easier to cater for than other groups. Generally their cardiovascular fitness needs to be increased, and the basic fitness components of strength, flexibility and muscular endurance can be improved as well. Attending classes with easy-to-follow fitness routines will allow beginners to keep up and enhance their skills almost immediately. A basic low-impact class with a caring and understanding instructor will be a good start to any beginner fitness regime.

Children

Children are increasingly becoming involved in fitness classes. Fitness classes for children are extremely important for a number of reasons, including:

- Low levels of Physical Education training and sport education in many schools
- Increasing concern about the number of overweight and obese children and adolescents
- Increasing evidence of poor diet and exercise regimes.

Unfortunately, few health and fitness centres offer programs for the young. While weight training for children and younger teenagers is not recommended, fitness/aerobics programs are a great way of ensuring suitable exercise for this group.

Owners and managers of fitness centres should expand their timetables to include specific classes for younger children and teenagers. Instructors need to increase their knowledge of children's fitness. Teachers need to promote extracurricular activities while parents should encourage their children to be more active, especially where children are not actively involved in organised sport or other physical activities such as dance or physical culture.

Different age groups require very different exercise formats.

3–5 years: 30 minutes

Simple, easy-to-follow warm-up using a game or simple aerobic moves. No more than three moves should be used in any aerobic sequence—for example, step touch, flick kick and grapevine. These moves are easily described with word and action—for example, when completing a flick kick emphasise flicking your boot off or kicking a football.

Other components of the class should include stretching and shapes: arch position, push-up position, straddle sit, etc., and simple skills including log rolls (sideways rolling), forward rolls, bunny hops (a tuck movement halfway to handstand), the sorts of things done in a Gymbaroo class.

To conclude the class teach a simple routine, perhaps something which combines movements like marching, jumping and bobbing.

6–13 years: 45 to 60 minutes

Easy-to-follow warm-ups with each lesson adding, linking and combining movements taught previously to make routines or sequences.

Fun, active games using the maximum-participation concept (no elimination or standing still at any one time).

Stretching, even learning to do the splits.

An aerobics routine where the children suggest movements they would like to put together into a sequence. This can be practised many times over to increase cardiovascular endurance.

Circuits are a great idea to keep children moving and on task. Depending on how many children are in the class, the groups working the circuit can contain up to five individuals.

The following is an example of a circuit:

Station:

1	Skipping with rope
2	Star jumps
3	Abdominal curls
4	Flick kicks
5	Weave-running laps around cones
6	Push-ups on knees and with straight back
7	Grapevines
8	Superman position (lying on the stomach with legs and arms in the air)
9	Standing long jumps up and down the room
10	Trampoline running

Participants can spend 30, 45 or 60 seconds at each station. They complete the circuit once, recording their repetitions, then do it again, trying to better their scores and competing against themselves.

The class could finish off with a routine that incorporates a theme—for example, use 'YMCA' (Village People) and get the children to do the actions on the chorus.

13 years and over: 45–60 minutes
This type of class is fun and rewarding. Begin with a warm-up, then a high and low impact with simple aerobic movements; each week you can add the movements together to make combinations and mini-routines. The main aim is to keep the cardiovascular section going for at least 20 minutes. A circuit similar to the one suggested for the 6–13 age group can be used, with the movements made harder—for example, changing the 'knee' push-ups to a full

position on the toes. Keep this section going for at least 15 or 20 minutes. This makes a 40-minute cardiovascular section, which should be enough to increase fitness when performed three times per week.

Conclude the class with some strength and muscle-conditioning exercises—abdominal work, back arches and push-ups should all be used. Try to reinforce good technique. Work on strengthening all abdominal muscles, especially those for posture.

Intellectually and physically disabled participants
Individuals with cerebral palsy, spinal injuries, or intellectual disabilities, and amputees can all benefit from some form of aerobic exercise. Detailed exercise routines to cover the needs of these groups fully is beyond the scope of this book.

MOTIVATION
Understanding aerobic exercise, its benefits, correct techniques and appropriate implementation is the basis of maintaining fitness; without acting on this understanding, nothing will be achieved. Consistent training is important—fitness will only remain or improve if exercise is maintained at a steady and achievable rate. To do this requires motivation. People are motivated by different things which depend on what is important to the individual, either psychologically and/or physically. Factors that commonly motivate people to exercise include the desire to win sporting events, the desire to improve appearance, control weight, boost energy levels and increase stamina; the wish to feel physically good, to increase strength, mental alertness and longevity; to increase general health and disease resistance, to improve mobility, to participate in specific activities such as a marathon.

APPENDIX I

ENERGY

- Energy is defined as the capacity to do work.
- Work is defined as the transferring of a force over a distance (i.e. work = force × distance).
- Power is defined as a measure of work carried out per unit of time.
- Efficiency = Work output × 100/Energy input.

Units of measurement
- *Work* and *power* are measured as work per unit of time (e.g. kilopond metre per minute or watts). Note: *kilopond* refers to the same unit of work as *kilogram-force*.
- Energy is expressed as k/cal or calories (1 k/cal = 1000 calories) *or* kilojoules *or* litres of oxygen per minute (generally 1 L/ O_2/min = 5 k/cal; this can vary).

THE NATURE OF ENERGY

- Energy can not be created or destroyed—it simply changes form.
- All energy in a person's body is ultimately derived from solar energy.
- Chemical energy is an important form of energy for human life.

ENERGY PRODUCTION PATHWAYS FROM DIFFERENT FOODS

Fats (triglycerides in the body)
- Hydrolysis of triglycerides produces glycerol and FFA.
- Beta-oxidation of glycerol produces acetyl CoA.

Carbohydrates
- Carbohydrates break down to glucose (simple sugar).
- Glycolysis of simple sugars produces pyruvic acid.
- Pyruvic acid produces acetyl CoA.

Proteins
- Proteins break down into amino acids.
- Deamination may occasionally occur to produce keto-acid.

MITOCHONDRIA

These are structures found inside cells, and are critical to aerobic capacity. Within the mitochondria, carbohydrates, fats and proteins are broken down to produce energy. The more mitochondria the better the endurance performance.

Research has shown:

- When levels of key hormones increase in the endocrine system, mitochondrial size and density increase, thus increasing aerobic capacity
- Regular exercise can increase the numbers of mitochondria
- The concentration of cytochrome (a key chemical found in mitochondria) increases with regular and appropriate levels of exercise.

APPENDIX II

THE SKELETAL SYSTEM

The bones of the body are connected by the joints into a framework called the skeleton. The skeleton carries out several important functions, the most important of which are:

- Providing **protection** to the vital organs of the body. For example, the brain is protected by the skull, while the remainder of the central nervous system (the spinal cord) is protected by the vertebral column or backbone. The ribcage protects the heart and lungs while the pelvic girdle covers the urogenital system.
- Providing the basis of the **general structure** and outline of the human body. It is the frame to which muscles and skin are attached.
- Giving the body **rigidity**.
- Acting as **levers** so that movements like walking, running and lifting can be performed.
- Providing a **storage site** for minerals, particularly calcium, phosphorus and magnesium. These are stored within the bones, and are utilised when they are deficient in the diet.
- Producing **marrow**, which plays a part in the formation of **blood cells** (mainly red blood cells but also some of the white blood cells).

Bones are living structures. They have blood vessels, lymphatic vessels and nerves. They grow, are able to repair themselves and are subject to diseases.

Bones are connected in a system of movable and immovable joints to form the skeleton. The skeleton serves as a frame to which vol-untary striated muscles are attached.

The skeletal system consists of bone tissue, cartilage, bone marrow, and the periosteum, the membrane surrounding the bones.

BONE ANATOMY

A typical long bone has a shaft and two ends (the extremities). The outer shell of a typical bone is made of compact bone, a hard layer which covers most of the surface. The two extremities consist of spongy bone, made up of fine plates forming a porous network. The spaces within this network are usually filled with bone marrow, a soft, fatty substance. Inside the shaft is the medullary cavity, a hollow also filled with bone marrow.

Some bone ends are involved in joint movement. Where this occurs the extremity is covered with a thin layer of smooth cartilage called the articular cartilage. Its job is to provide a friction-free surface to aid movement.

Around the entire surface of the bone (except where there is articular cartilage) is a thin, fibrous membrane called the periosteum. The bone-forming cells (osteoblasts) located here are responsible for laying down bone to increase the width of long bones. The periosteum also lays down bone as a healing response at places where fractures have occurred.

Between the shaft and the extremity is a disc of cartilage called the epiphysial cartilage. Osteoblasts located in this disc lay down bone which makes the bone longer. This disc is only active until mature size is reached, after which the disc ossifies. In humans bone maturity occurs in the late teens or early twenties.

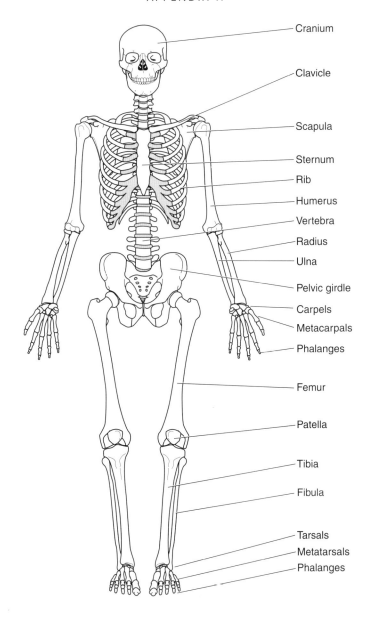

Cranium

Clavicle

Scapula

Sternum

Rib

Humerus

Vertebra

Radius

Ulna

Pelvic girdle

Carpels

Metacarpals

Phalanges

Femur

Patella

Tibia

Fibula

Tarsals

Metatarsals

Phalanges

About one-third of the weight of bone consists a framework of fibrous tissues and cells. The other two-thirds of the weight comes from the inorganic salts which are deposited within the framework to make bone tissue hard. These salts are chiefly (some 80 per cent) calcium and phosphorus as calcium phosphate. Other salts include calcium carbonate and magnesium phosphate.

JOINTS

Bones are joined to one another by joints of several types.

Immoveable Good examples of immovable joints are those of the skull. The skull bones cannot move after maturity due to ossification of the connecting tissues.

Slightly moveable This sort of joint is

found between the vertebrae of the spine.

Freely moveable Knee and wrist joints are examples of freely moveable joints. A joint does not have to be able to move in all directions to be termed freely moveable. It might move in all directions (like the shoulder joint) or in one plane only (like the knee joint).

The freely moveable joint is encased by the joint capsule which consists of an outer fibrous ligament which is thick and strong and an inner synovial membrane which is thin and delicate. This membrane secretes synovial fluid ('joint oil') to lubricate the joint. The surfaces of the bones involved in movement are covered by the very smooth articular cartilage which assists movement.

BONE MOVEMENTS

Bones are enabled to move by a three-part process:

1. Contraction of a muscle attached to two different bones
2. One end of the muscle is attached to a bone which remains still, the other end to a different bone which is able to move
3. A nerve stimulates selected muscle tissue to contract, drawing together the two bones to which that muscle is attached.

JOINT DAMAGE

Joints can be damaged by the activity a person performs. Running over rough terrain, netball and other sports requiring quick stop/go or impact movements can cause serious damage to the components of joints, bones and ligaments. Degenerative diseases like arthritis will also cause inflammation and reduction of the joint's mobility.

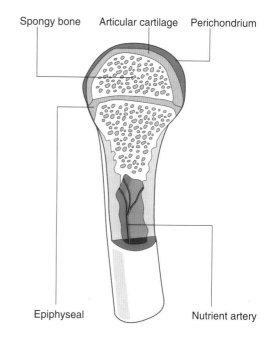

Spongy bone　　Articular cartilage　　Perichondrium

Epiphyseal　　　　　　　　　　Nutrient artery

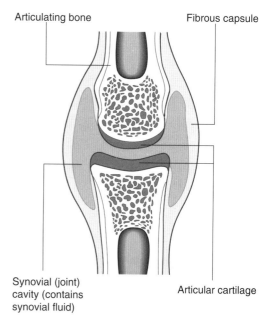

Articulating bone　　　　　　Fibrous capsule

Synovial (joint) cavity (contains synovial fluid)　　　　Articular cartilage

APPENDIX III

DESIGNING FITNESS TESTS

When you make a decision about what tests to use or not use in assessing fitness (Chapter 6), the following criteria need to be considered.

VALIDITY

This is the degree to which the test determines the characteristic of fitness which it is intended to indicate.

Example: If it provides a strong indication of aerobic fitness, then it is highly valid. If it only provides a general indication of aerobic fitness, it may need to be used in conjunction with other tests for aerobic fitness to provide a cumulative indication with adequate validity.

RELIABILITY

This is the degree to which a fitness test is able to measure a particular factor. A test may be reliable (measuring a factor well), but not valid because it is measuring something which is not particularly relevant to what the fitness testing is intended to achieved.

OBJECTIVITY

This is the degree to which results are consistent with respect to the quality of performance by persons undertaking a particular fitness test. Tests such as measuring weight, the height a person can jump, or distances stretched in a flexibility test, tend to be objective—that is, consistent with a person's capabilities—hence they reflect fitness.

A test such as swimming, however, may lose objectivity if conducted under various swimming conditions (swimming in the ocean, where one is affected by waves and currents, may well give different results from swimming in an Olympic pool). Water temperature is also important. If a test is conducted in extremely cold conditions the body takes longer to warm up and the nervous system does not function to its maximum. Body fat percentage tests performed by different fitness can vary slightly in method, giving skewed results.

ADMINISTRATIVE USEABILITY

This refers to the ability of the test to provide useable information.

RECOMMENDED PROCEDURE FOR CONSTRUCTING A NEW FITNESS TEST SERIES*

1. Determine what characteristics should be measured. Draw up a list with input from several experts.
2. Prepare test specifications for each listed characteristic. Include exact instructions of how scoring should be undertaken.
3. Trial proposed tests on a randomly selected sample group. For a major or important series of tests, where they are to be used on large numbers of people for a long period of time, a sample group of 200 would be appropriate.
4. Evaluate the results. Consider validity,

* Adapted from Bosco, J.S., and Gustafson, W.F., (1983), *Measurement and Evaluation in Physical Education, Fitness and Sports*, Prentice Hall, New Jersey

reliability, objectivity and administrative useability. Check on routine reliability errors; that is, whether the same results are achieved if the same test is conducted several times on the same person.

5. Study and determine the physical accuracy of each type of measurement. This may also involve testing the accuracy of measuring equipment and specifying how to calibrate, use and/or maintain equipment in future tests.

6. Conduct a statistical analysis of test results to help identify any deviations or discrepancies.

7. Determine expected scores for different demographic groupings such as different levels of fitness (beginners, average and advanced); different sexes; different ages.

8. Adjust test configuration if necessary to improve the series.

APPENDIX IV

DEALING WITH COMPLAINTS

Research has often shown that only a minor proportion of dissatisfied clients or customers actually lodge a complaint with a business.* In light of this, it is reasonable to assume that one complaint made may well indicate several dissatisfied people. Conversely, a dissatisfied customer will often complain to other customers, thus tending to spread ill-will towards the business.

Managers and instructors should make a constant effort to identify dissatisfied customers before their dissatisfaction becomes a problem, particularly the silent majority who do not complain. If these people can be identified before they depart a facility or service you have an opportunity to deal with the problem, regain their confidence, and retain them as patrons. Effective and consistent communication with customers is very important! Identifying the dissatisfied customer who does not complain may be done in a number of different ways:

- Use regular questionnaires, inviting customers to write down any suggestions for improving your service. People who won't complain in person may raise issues of concern at one remove on a questionnaire.
- Talk to patrons frequently, and ask how you can help them more. If you are relaxed in your approach, they will be more relaxed about giving a truthful response.

* Manning, G.L., and Reece, B.L. (1989), *Selling Today*, Prentice Hall, New Jersey

- Keep track of patronage. Keep good records of when specific patrons use your services; and analyse the records to determine any changes in a client's pattern of usage. If there is a negative trend, ask why, in a relaxed way—don't intimidate!
- When a customer talks—listen. Hear what people say, remember it, write it down, analyse it. Don't dominate a conversation when someone is trying to express discontent.
- Don't make excuses! Never try to pass the buck. It is tempting to attribute blame in the face of criticism, but a customer will respond far better to a positive comment: 'Thanks for letting us know; we'll try to do something about that straight away.' You can politely explain the reasons why things are the way they are, but try to do it in a positive way.

Remember

Although there may be a cost involved in satisfying a disgruntled customer, there can be a far greater cost involved in losing that customer. Extra promotion will be required to replace the customer; worse, extra work may be required to counteract the negative publicity coming from a dissatisfied former customer telling friends what they think about you. A customer lost is more than lost business from one person. Anyone who abandons a service or organisation due to a perceived disservice will tell many other people of their dissatisfaction.

APPENDIX V

COURSE DIRECTORY

A wide range of health and fitness courses has been developed for distance education by the author of this book and staff at the Australian Correspondence Schools. These include short courses (for anyone wishing to improve their own health and fitness), through to full professional training in the areas of fitness and recreation.

Short courses include:
Aerobics
Health and Wellbeing
Advanced Aerobics
Health and Fitness
Human Nutrition
Fitness
Fitness Risk Management
Recreation Management
Recreation Marketing
Recreation Facilities
Aquafitness
Resistance and Gym Supervision
Psychology and Counselling
Aromatherapy
Human Biology

Accredited training courses at the time of publication include:
Fitness Leaders Certificate
Advanced Diploma in Recreation—Fitness

plus many more. All certificates and diplomas are internationally accredited with the International Accreditation and Recognition Council.

Videos
Through the school the author has also produced a range of videos in fitness and other disciplines.

Handbook
For a free copy of the school's handbook or video list, contact:

Australian Correspondence Schools
PO Box 2092, Nerang MDC, Qld 4211
Ph: (07) 5530 4855, Fax: (07) 5525 1728

Also at:
264 Swansea Rd, Lilydale, Vic 3140
Ph: (03) 9736 1882, Fax: (03) 9736 4034

The school can be e-mailed at:
    admin@acs.edu.au
or   acs@onthe.net.au

Further details on the school's courses, as well as careers advice, and other information, can be found on the following Internet sites:
    http://www.acs.edu.au
or   http://www.acs.edu.au/recnfit

APPENDIX VI

EQUIPMENT SUPPLIERS

Aerobic Microphones Aust P/L
Microphones for aerobic and aqua-aerobic instructors.
PO Box 321, Alexandria, NSW 2015
Ph: (02) 9313 4995, Fax: (02) 9313 5569

Australian Barbell Co.
Weights, aerobic equipment.
54 Bond St West, Mordialloc, Vic 3195
Ph: (03) 9580 5945, Fax: (03) 9580 3656

Calgym Equipment
Cardiovascular exercise equipment.
PO Box 129, Ashmore City, Qld 4214
Ph: 0500 536 968, Fax: 0500 536 969

Cybex
Resistance and cardiovascular fitness equipment.
7 Dickson Ave, Artarmon, NSW 2064
Ph: (02) 9906 2211, Fax: (02) 9906 2090

H F Industries
PO Box 2221, Taren Point, NSW 2229
Ph: (02) 9531 6700, Fax: (02) 9531 6722

Keylink Physical Care P/L
Fitness equipment, including steppers, rowers, stationary bikes and treadmills.
335 Prospect Rd, Blair Athol, SA 5084
Ph: (08) 8260 5633, Fax: (08) 8349 6599

Muscleworks Bodybuilding & Fitness Equipment
Fitness equipment and clothing manufacturers & distributors.
Shops 3 & 4
433 Nepean Hwy, Frankston, Vic 3199
Ph: (03) 9781 1311, Fax: (03) 9770 1923

No Fear
Fitness, sport and leisure wear.

2 Perkins Place, Torquay, Vic. 3228
Ph: (03) 5261 6366, Fax: (03) 5261 6461

Olympic Fitness Equipment
Resistance and cardiovascular exercise equipment.
660 Whitehorse Rd, Mitcham, Vic 3132
Ph: (03) 9874 6888, Fax: (03) 9873 3705

Only Fitness (Aust) P/L
Fitness equipment.
9 Tandem Ave, Kawana Waters, Qld 4575
Ph: (07) 5493 7317, Fax: (07) 5493 7387

Powertec Fitness Equipment P/L
Resistance and cardiovascular exercise equipment.
PO Box 982, Neutral Bay, NSW 2089
Ph: (02) 9908 4064, Fax: (02) 9904 4680

PR Medical P/L
Australian supplier of body composition analysers for measuring fat percentage.
PO Box 608, Everton Park, Qld 4053
Ph: (07) 3353 1599, Fax: (07) 3353 1592

Quirks Quatics
Deep-water running belts
20 Stones Court, Tallebudgera Valley, Qld 4228
Ph: (07) 5533 8368

Rival Swimwear
Unit 10, 26–34 Dunning Ave, Rosebery, NSW 2018
Ph: (02) 9663 2111, Fax: (02) 9663 2122

Running Bare Aust. P/L
Aerobic, training and leisure wear.
City South Business Park
Unit 10, 26–34 Dunning Ave, Rosebery, NSW 2018
Ph: (02) 9663 2111, Fax: (02) 9663 2122

Sterns Playland P/L
Resistance and cardiovascular fitness equipment.
PO Box 120, Miller, NSW 2168
Ph: (02) 9608 1111, Fax: (02) 9608 1022

Vector Fitness Products
PO Box 611, Willunga, SA 5172
Ph/Fax: (08) 8326 8400

Workout Workshop
Gymnasium and fitness equipment.
2–4 Cochranes Rd, Moorabbin, Vic. 3189
Ph: (03) 9553 3153, Fax: (03) 9555 0375

York Fitness Aust.
Resistance and cardiovascular exercise equipment.
Lot 1/Unit 2 Swaffham Rd, Minto, NSW 2566
Ph: (02) 9603 8444, Fax: (02) 9603 8555

APPENDIX VII

FITNESS-RELATED MAGAZINES

Australian Cyclist Magazine
PO Box 344, Berry, NSW 2533
Ph/Fax: (02) 4464 3255

Australian Swimming & Fitness
PO Box 2805, Taren Point, NSW 2229
Ph: (02) 9542 7335, (02) 9542 7323

Australian Triathlete
PO Box 19, Armadale, Vic. 3143
Ph: (03) 9822 3099, Fax: (03) 9822 8345

Fitness Australia
Full coverage of fitness-related topics.
PO Box 4075 Mulgrave, Vic. 3170
Ph: (03) 9574 8999, Fax: (03) 9574 8899

Fun Runner Magazine
PO Box 2805, Taren Point, NSW 2229
Ph: (02) 9544 6366, Fax: (02) 9544 6220

Sports Health & The Australian Journal of
Science and Medicine in Sport
PO Box 897, Belconnen, ACT 2616
Ph: (02) 6251 6944, Fax: (02) 6253 1489

Sports Med News
*Official journal of Sports Medicine Australia,
Queensland Branch.*
PO Box 240, St Lucia, Qld 4067
Ph: (07) 3870 4195, Fax: (07) 3870 7584

Triathlon Sports Magazine
PO Box 2805, Taren Point, NSW 2229
Ph: (02) 9542 7335, Fax: (02) 9542 7323

Ultra-Fit Magazine
PO Box 880, Newport Beach, NSW 2106
Ph: (02) 9999 3384, Fax: (02) 9999 3385

APPENDIX VIII

FITNESS ORGANISATIONS

Australia
Aerokid
Children and Youth Health and Fitness
Promotes and specialises in aerobics/fitness
workshops and books for children/teenagers.
47 Oaktree Rd, North Croydon, Vic. 3136
Ph: (03) 9723 1005

Australian Council of Health, Physical
Education and Recreation (ACHPER)
214 Port Rd, Hindmarsh, SA 5007
Ph: (08) 8340 3388
Publish a variety of magazines including:
ACHPER Catalogue (purchasing information for
equipment)
ACHPER Healthy Lifestyles
Active and Healthy Quarterly

Australian Fitness Accreditation Council
(AFAC)
GPO Box 2018, Canberra City, ACT 2601
Ph: (0416) 207 847

Australian Gymnastics Federation (AGF)
Specialising in sport aerobics for competitions.
647 Burwood Rd, Hawthorn, Vic. 3123
Ph: (03) 9882 3111 Fax: (03) 9882 3325
E-mail address: ausgymsport.gov.au

Fitlink Australia
PO Box 1134, Coorparoo DC, Qld 4151
Ph: (07) 3393 0977, Fax: (07) 3393 0829

Fitnation
Level 19 Como Business Centre,
644 Chapel St, South Yarra, Vic. 3141
Phone: (03) 9823 6290, Fax: (03) 9826 3642

Fitness Australia Association Inc.
GPO Box 2018, Canberra City, ACT 2601
Ph: (02) 6230 1989

'Motive 8'—Music for Fitness Professionals
PO Box 351, Warrandyte, Vic. 3113
Ph: (03) 9844 1964, Fax: (03) 9844 1978

Network
Publishes a variety of fitness-related magazines and
newsletters.
PO Box 57, Neutral Bay, NSW 2089
Ph: (02) 9908 4944, Fax: (02) 9908 4349

International
Federation Internationale de Sport, Aerobics et
Fitness (FISAF)
PO Box 378, Wollongong East, NSW 2500
Ph: (02) 4227 1575, Fax: (02) 4229 3486

INDEX